Nursing in the Coronary Care Unit

Nursing in the Coronary Care Unit

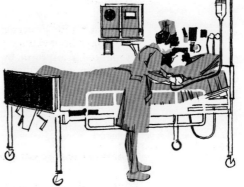

LaVaughn Sharp, R.N., M.A.
Director, School of Nursing,
The Grace Hospital, Medical Center,
Detroit, Michigan

Beatrice Rabin, R.N.
Supervisor, Coronary Care Unit and Intensive Care Unit,
The Grace Hospital, Northwest Unit,
Detroit, Michigan

5405

J. B. Lippincott Company   Philadelphia • Toronto

Distributed in Great Britain by
Blackwell Scientific Publications, Oxford and Edinburgh

Library of Congress Catalog Card Number 74-124095

Printed in the United States of America

PREFACE

To reduce the mortality rate resulting from the complications of acute myocardial infarction a coronary care unit must be available in every hospital and clinic across the country.

The nurses who staff these units must be knowledgeable in the care of the coronary patient and be prepared to make decisions to initiate appropriate measures. The need for an organized educational program to teach nurses to function with a specialized competence in the field of coronary care nursing is essential if the nursing profession is to help meet one of the major health problems in the nation.

This book is designed to enlarge the nursing student's understanding of the coronary care concept. It should prove a valuable source of information for the nurse specialist practicing in this area. It is also directed to nursing service administrators who must initiate the establishment of a coronary care unit and are concerned with setting up an in-service educational program in order to maintain a qualified staff.

In every real sense this book demonstrates the cooperative efforts of administration, nursing education, nursing service and the cardiology staff to establish two coronary care units at the Grace Hospital in Detroit, Michigan.

We wish to thank Dr. Roger DeBusk, Director of the Grace Hospital, who made available all hospital facilities, and Mr. William Loechel, Medical Illustrator at Wayne State University College of Medicine, whose illustrations enhance the presentation of the material.

We wish to thank Mr. Joseph Lipiec, biomedical representative for the General Electric Company, for permission to photograph the monitoring equipment, and a special thanks to Dr. Carlos Augusto Godoy, Medical

Resident, who demonstrated the use of this equipment for the photographs.

We are grateful to Dr. H. S. Mellen, F.A.C.P., and Dr. Stanley Wolfe, members of the Grace Hospital Cardiology Staff, who reviewed Chapters 8, 9, 10 and 11 for medical accuracy, and assisted in the selection of the oscilloscope tracings for presentation.

A special thanks is due Dr. Floyd Levagood, F.A.C.P., who reviewed the manuscript, and to Mr. Donald Yarnevic, M.A., Assistant Professor of Philosophy at Mercy College of Detroit, who assisted in the formulation of philosophical principles and who offered many suggestions regarding the style of the presentation.

Finally, we wish to thank the J. B. Lippincott Company, Mr. David Miller, Editorial Manager of the Nursing Department, and Miss Mary Dennesaites, Associate Editor, Nursing Department, for their expert guidance and counsel in the completion of this work.

LaVaughn Sharp
Beatrice Rabin

CONTENTS

INTRODUCTION

The electronic revolution in America that provided the capability to place man on the moon has invaded the modern hospital to assist the medical and nursing professions to eliminate the great plague of the 20th century—coronary artery disease.

Eight years ago a new concept of treatment—the coronary care unit—challenged nurses to use the resuscitative techniques necessary to reverse a catastrophic arrhythmia. Today, the chief objective is to prevent the need for resuscitation. Monitoring instruments, which make possible the constant, visual observation of the cardiac cycle, allow for the recognition and treatment of minor arrhythmias and thus help to prevent the development of a major disorganization of the electromotive forces of the heart.

It is to this intent that the following objectives for this text are established:

1. To present the concepts and principles necessary to understand the function and the pathology of the circulatory system
2. To present the most common diagnostic tests used to confirm the diagnosis of acute myocardial infarction
3. To present the significant clinical manifestations of coronary artery disorders, including their etiology and complications, as well as the treatment and the nursing intervention necessary to implement the principles involved in the care of the patient with a myocardial infarction

Effective nursing care in cardiac conditions requires a thorough knowledge of the pathologic and physiologic processes that are involved. To guide the professional nurse in understanding the principles and diagnostic measures used in the care of patients with coronary artery disease, the normal anatomy and physiology of the heart are reviewed in Chapter 1.

Chapter 2 outlines the diagnostic procedures used to establish the

1

diagnosis of a cardiac condition, and the etiology and complications of coronary artery disease are discussed in Chapter 3.

To develop and maintain high standards of patient care, the coronary care unit must be well organized. Responsibilities must be delegated so that preventive or therapeutic measures may be carried out quickly by trained personnel. Chapters 4 and 5 on the organization of the coronary care unit provide guidance both for the establishment as well as the use of such a specialized facility.

In order that the correct emphasis be given the *total* treatment of the cardiac patient, Chapter 6, Psychological Responses in the Coronary Care Unit, deals with the nurse-patient relationship and patient rehabilitation, preceding those chapters that deal with medical aspects.

The nurse in the coronary care unit must be able to carry out emergency procedures. She must therefore be well trained, confident, and duly authorized to act. To enhance the nurse's knowledge of emergency situations, Chapter 7 deals with the complications which may occur with myocardial infarctions.

To carry out her most important function—prompt intervention—the nurse in the coronary care unit must be able to make correct electrocardiographic interpretations of cardiac arrhythmias. She must therefore have a thorough knowledge of the electrical basis of cardiac monitoring (Chap. 8). The basic concepts of arrhythmias are discussed in Chapter 9, and disorders of impulse formation and of impulse conduction in Chapters 10 and 11.

Care of the patient with a pacemaker is discussed in Chapter 12.

The nurse must also be well trained in relevant clinical pharmacology. The drugs used in the coronary care unit are discussed in Chapter 13.

Recognizing the need for extending fully professional coronary care, the final chapter presents a plan for initiating an in-service educational program directed toward the development and maintenance of a highly competent staff of cardiac nurse-specialists.

1 NORMAL ANATOMY AND PHYSIOLOGY OF THE HEART

This chapter is presented as a brief review to augment the nurse's knowledge of the normal anatomy and physiology of the heart.

The circulatory system is designed to deliver blood to and from the capillaries, where the blood gives up its oxygen and takes in carbon dioxide and other waste products. Some of the fluid portion of the blood leaves the vessels to provide tissue nourishment; this tissue fluid then drains into blood capillaries and lymphatic capillaries as it begins its journey back to the heart.

The center of the circulatory system is the heart, a hollow, muscular contractile organ. Its only function is to pump blood continuously throughout the body in a closed system of vessels.

Blood returns from all parts of the body, except the lungs, via the superior and inferior venae cavae, which open into the right atrium, from which the blood is pumped through the tricuspid valve and into the right ventricle.

Beginning at the left side, Figure 1–1 shows the right side of the heart where the transportation function of the circulatory system begins. Blood leaves the right ventricle via the pulmonary artery to the lungs for oxygenation. It then leaves the lungs via the pulmonary veins to enter the left atrium, then to the left ventricle, which ejects the blood into the aorta.

Circulation is vital in maintaining a constant internal environment: the blood carries food and oxygen to the tissues; waste products are carried from the tissues to the organs of excretion.

By its rapid circulation, the blood regulates body temperature. It transports hormones, produced by the endocrine glands, which regulate metabolism. It helps maintain the proper acid-base balance of the cells. It aids in the body's defense against invading organisms by the action of the white blood cells and antibodies it contains.

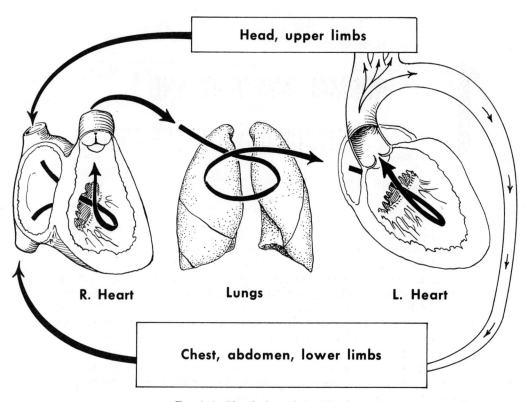

FIG. 1–1. Circulation of the blood.

The heart, composed chiefly of muscle, is a double pump which operates continuously due to the properties of the heart muscle.

Automaticity is the ability of the heart cells to regularly discharge the inherent electrical impulse initiating contraction of the heart. Normally, automaticity is greatest in the S-A (sino-atrial) node, and the rate of impulse generated at this site determines the cardiac rate.

Rhythmicity is the cardiac muscle's inherent ability to contract rhythmically, though its rhythm is modified by the autonomic nervous system.

Conductivity is the ability of the heart tissue to transmit electrical impulses, regardless of where the impulses generate. Heart structures especially conductive are the A-V (atrio-ventricular) node, the A-V bundle and the Purkinje fibers. Coordinated cardiac contraction requires a system which distributes the electrical impulse to the muscle fibers of the atria and ventricles in the proper sequence and time. The speed of conduction is as follows:

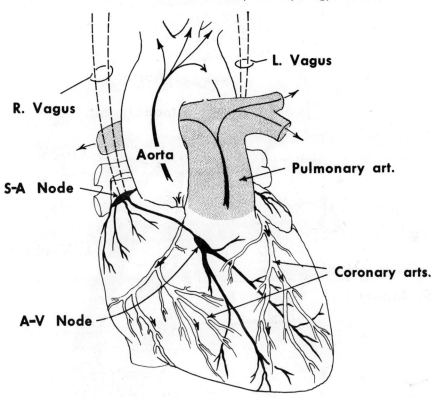

FIG. 1–2. External view of the heart.

Atrial muscle—1000 mm./sec.
Ventricular muscle—400 mm./sec.
Purkinje fibers—4000 mm./sec.
Atrio-ventricular junction—200 mm./sec.[1]

The external view of the heart in Figure 1–2 displays the relationships of the heart chambers, the major blood vessels and nerve supply. The heart is supplied with two sets of motor nerve fibers. The parasympathetic fibers reach the heart through the vagus nerves. Nerve impulses over these fibers decrease the rate of impulse formation by the S-A node, and are called inhibitory. Impulses over the sympathetic fibers are called accelerators because they cause the heart to beat faster and harder in stressful situations.

[1] Stock, J. P. P.: Diagnosis and Treatment of Cardiac Arrhythmias. p. 9. New York, Appleton-Century-Crofts, 1969.

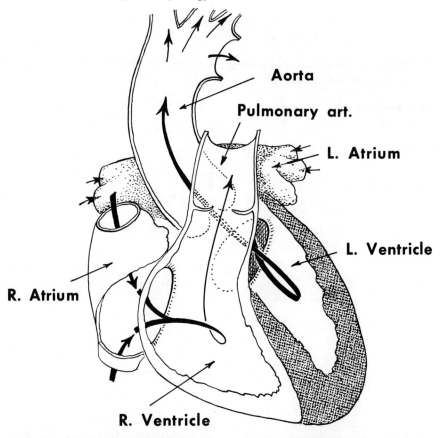

FIG. 1–3. Relationship of the heart's chambers and valves.

Figure 1–3 shows the flow of blood through the chambers and valves in the heart. The right atrium receives venous blood from all parts of the body except the lungs, including venous drainage from the heart. The blood flows from the right atrium through the tricuspid valve into the right ventricle. During ventricular systole the blood pours through the pulmonary valve and the pulmonary artery to the lungs for oxygenation. Blood returns from the lungs through the pulmonary veins to the left atrium. It then passes through the mitral valve to the left ventricle. The left ventricle ejects blood through the aorta, located on its superior surface.

Note that the mitral valve prevents backflow of blood from ventricle to atrium during ventricular contraction. If the mitral valve flaps are damaged as a result of rheumatic fever, two conditions may result:

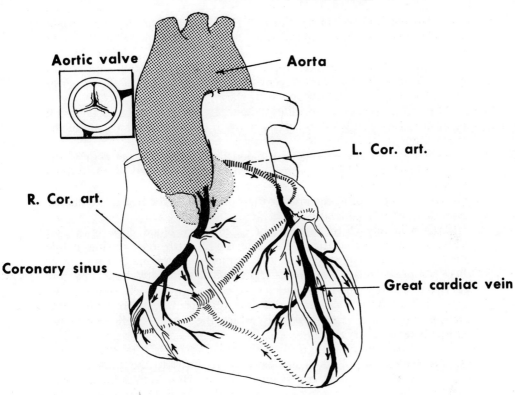

Aortic valve

Aorta

L. Cor. art.

R. Cor. art.

Coronary sinus

Great cardiac vein

FIG. 1–4. Coronary circulation.

1. Valvular stenosis
2. Valvular insufficiency

Mitral stenosis results in stasis in the pulmonary circulation, increasing the work of the right ventricle. Chronic congestion of the lungs and right ventricle hypertrophy usually accompany severe stenosis.

In the presence of aortic valve insufficiency, some of the blood ejected during ventricular systole leaks back into the ventricle during diastole. In order to meet the needs of the body, the heart must pump more blood than a normal heart. This compensatory measure results in progressive ventricular hypertrophy.

As blood leaves the left ventricle, part of it enters the left and right coronary arteries which nourish the heart (see Fig. 1–4). The left coronary artery divides into the left anterior descending artery and the left circumflex artery. The left anterior descending artery supplies the anterior surface of the left ventricle, the medial portion of the anterior surface of the right ventricle and the lower third of the posterior surface of the right ventricle. The remainder of the right ventricle is supplied by the right coronary artery.

The left circumflex artery supplies the lateral wall and the apical half of the posterior wall of the left ventricle. The upper half of the posterior wall of the left ventricle is supplied by the right coronary artery.

The coronary vessels are independent of each other; hence, if one of the arteries is suddenly occluded, no blood is delivered to that part of the myocardium which it supplies.

At rest the volume of coronary blood flow is about 4 per cent of the total cardiac output. While cardiac output can be increased up to 10 times its normal, the coronary blood flow can be increased only up to 6 times its normal. In other words, the greater the work load of the heart, the smaller the ratio of coronary blood flow.

Approximately 75 to 80 per cent of coronary blood flow to the left ventricle occurs during diastole. There is very little flow during systole due to the compression effect of the cardiac contraction. During systole there is more coronary flow to the right ventricle than to the left because the pressure within the right ventricle is less than in the left and the compression effect to the coronary of the right ventricle is less. All these factors become important in tachycardia, in which the total diastolic period per minute is significantly reduced.

Collateral circulation between the coronary arteries is extremely poor. Collateral blood supply does not exist in the heart to the extent that it exists in most tissues and organs of the body. However, there is a considerable degree of anastomosis between the terminal branches of the coronary arteries. This anastomosis increases rapidly when the blood supply to any area of the heart is threatened. It is these rapidly developing collateral channels that enable a patient to recover from the various types of coronary occlusions. However, the fact that the coronary arteries are end arteries with relatively few connections to nearby branches is the cause of thousands of deaths every year.

After the blood passes through the capillaries, it is collected by the cardiac veins; these empty into the coronary sinus, a short vein, located on the posterior side of the heart, which opens into the right atrium. Cardiac veins that do not empty into the coronary sinus, such as the anterior cardiac veins, empty into the right atrium. A few smaller veins empty into the ventricles.

Figure 1–5 accents the special neuromuscular tissues which are concerned with the electrical phenomena in the heart. The stimulus for the heartbeat arises in the S-A node, the pacemaker of the heart. The impulse spreads through the atria in all directions. This excitation wave results in the P wave of the electrocardiogram. During the atrial contraction that

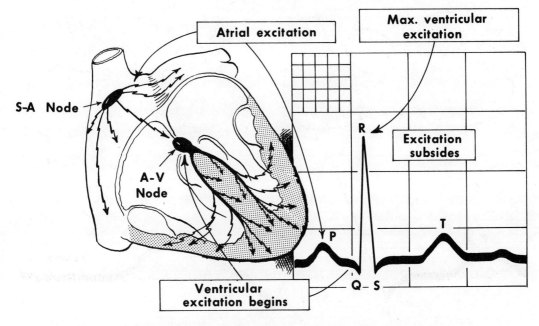

FIG. 1–5. Conduction system of the heart.

follows, the impulse reaches the A-V node, where it is delayed momentarily. It is then transmitted rapidly through the A-V node, and passes down the A-V bundle, the bundle branches, and the Purkinje fibers. These events are represented in the electrocardiogram by the P-R segment.

The electrical impulse spreads through the Purkinje system to the walls of the ventricles, resulting in ventricular contraction. This gives rise to the QRS complex of the ECG (electrocardiogram). Ventricular systole takes place between the peak of the QRS complex and the T wave, which occurs as ventricular excitation subsides.

The normal rate of impulse formation in the S-A node is 60–100 per minute, in the A-V node it is 40–60 per minute, and in the ventricles, 20–40 per minute. Under normal conditions, pacemaker activity may be taken over by the A-V node or the ventricles by increasing their rate above that of the S-A node, or by the S-A node's decreasing its rate below that of the others.

This can be demonstrated in the various arrhythmias. In junctional (nodal) tachycardia, the A-V node sends out impulses at a faster rate than the S-A node. In atrial fibrillation, the pacemaker is ectopic, being located in the atria. The atria quiver rather than contract and therefore are not under control of the S-A node.

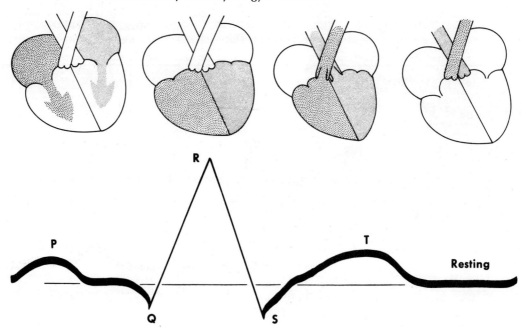

FIG. 1–6. Relationship between the cardiac cycle and the ECG.

Ventricular fibrillation is the result of an ectopic or irritable focus in the ventricles, and is incompatible with life since the ventricles no longer contract simultaneously. The chaotic ventricles cannot pump blood, and circulatory failure occurs. Death is imminent unless cardiac massage is instituted and maintained until electrical defibrillation can be performed. The electrical current from the defibrillator penetrates most of the fibers of the ventricles, stimulating all parts at the same time and causing them to become refractory. All impulses stop for 3 to 5 seconds, and if defibrillation is effective, a previous pacemaker in the S-A node, the atria or the ventricles will recapture the role of pacemaker.

Figure 1–6 shows the cardiac cycle and its relationship to the ECG. The cardiac cycle consists of three periods: systole, diastole, and a rest period. The cardiac cycle is initiated by depolarization of the S-A node, which initiates a depolarization wave which is propagated through the atria. The P wave is the result of atrial depolarization.

Blood enters the atria, and when the atrial pressure exceeds the pressure in the relaxed ventricles, the atrio-ventricular valves open and the blood flows into the ventricles.

The electrical stimulus arrives at the A-V node and spreads down the Purkinje system. This results in the QRS complex of the ECG. The ventricles contract. The A-V valves are closed and the pressure in the ventricles increases because of contraction. The aortic and pulmonic valves open and ventricular ejection occurs.

The ventricles relax. This results in the T wave of the ECG. The semilunar valves close. The atria fill with blood as ventricular diastole is being concluded.

The cardiac cycle is now complete. This entire sequence of events occurs during a single heartbeat in less than one second.

TABLE 1-1. EVENTS OF THE CARDIAC CYCLE

CONDUCTION	ECG	ATRIA	VALVES	VENTRICLES
S-A node impulse through atria to A-V node	P wave	Contract (depolarization)	A-V valves open, semilunar valves closed	Relaxed, fill with blood
Impulse from A-V node to A-V bundle, bundle branches, Purkinje system	QRS complex	Relaxed, fill with blood	A-V valves closed, semilunar valves open	Contract (depolarization), eject blood into aorta and pulmonary artery
	T wave			End of ventricular excitation; repolarization

REFERENCES AND BIBLIOGRAPHY

Bernreiter, M.: Electrocardiography. ed. 2. Philadelphia, J. B. Lippincott, 1963.

Chaffee, E. E., and Greisheimer, E. C.: Basic Physiology and Anatomy. ed. 2. Philadelphia, J. B. Lippincott, 1969.

Crouch, J. E.: Fundamental Human Anatomy. Philadelphia, Lea & Febiger, 1965.

Goss, C. M.: Gray's Anatomy of the Human Body. ed. 28. Philadelphia, Lea & Febiger, 1966.

Guyton, A. C.: Textbook of Medical Physiology. ed. 3. Philadelphia, W. B. Saunders, 1966.

Kimber, D. C., and Gray, C. E., et al: Anatomy and Physiology. ed. 15. New York, Macmillan, 1966.

Stock, J. P. P.: Diagnosis and Treatment of Cardiac Arrhythmias. New York, Appleton-Century-Crofts, 1969.

Tuttle, W. W., and Schottelius, B. A.: Textbook of Physiology. ed. 15. St. Louis, C. V. Mosby, 1965.

2 DIAGNOSTIC PROCEDURES

THE PATIENT'S HISTORY

In most instances the patient experiences and describes the sudden onset of persistent, severe, oppressive, substernal pain. This is followed by dyspnea, profuse diaphoresis, weakness, nausea, possible vomiting and extreme apprehension.

During physical examination, the patient appears to be in acute distress, with symptoms of shock such as cyanosis, pale, clammy skin, rapid, weak pulse and hypotension. Complications of infarction may include congestive heart failure and an arrhythmia.

Within 24 to 48 hours a moderate fever develops along with leukocytosis, an elevated sedimentation rate and transaminase. Electrocardiographic changes generally appear within 2 hours.

LABORATORY TESTS

Blood Analysis

COMPLETE BLOOD COUNT (CBC)

The red blood cells, or **erythrocytes**, carry oxygen to the tissues, carry carbon dioxide from the tissues, and help maintain the normal acid-base balance.

The measurement of the number of red blood cells, normally approximately 4.5 to 5.5 million per cu. mm. of blood, and the amount of hemoglobin, normally about 15 Gm. per 100 ml. of whole blood, are important because so many diseases are complicated by anemia. A low hemoglobin frequently occurs in bacterial endocarditis, rheumatic heart disease and the anemias. An increase in erythrocytes occurs in some types of chronic heart disease as well as in some congenital heart defects and polycythemia.

The white blood cells, or **leukocytes,** defend the body against invading microorganisms. An increase in number, normally 5,000 to 10,000 per cu. mm. of whole blood, is seen in infections, myocardial infarction and rheumatic heart disease.

WHITE CELL DIFFERENTIAL COUNT

The **neutrophils** ingest bacteria, and constitute from 54 to 62 per cent of the total number of leukocytes. The number of neutrophils is increased with infection, diabetic acidosis and coronary occlusion.

The **monocytes** function well as phagocytes, and constitute from 3 to 7 per cent of the leukocytes. An increase in the number of monocytes is frequent in subacute bacterial endocarditis.

The **lymphocytes** are concerned with the formation of antibodies, and form from 25 to 35 per cent of the leukocytes. An increase occurs with acute infections.

The **eosinophils** give evidence of adrenal function, and make up 1 to 3 per cent of the leukocytes. A decrease is noted in shock, severe infection and congestive heart failure.

The **basophils** constitute 0.5 to 1 per cent of the leukocytes, and increase in number during the healing process of inflammation.

ERYTHROCYTE SEDIMENTATION RATE

The normal ESR is 1.0 to 20 mm. per hour. It is increased in various infections, heart disease, acute bacterial endocarditis, coronary thrombosis, myocardial infarction and frequently in malignancies. The increase is noted within 2 or 3 days after the infarction and slowly decreases until the infarct is healed.

COAGULATION TIME

The Lee-White bleeding time is 5 to 8 minutes; the Duke method is 1 to 5 minutes. It is increased in anticoagulant therapy employing heparin.

PROTHROMBIN TIME

The prothrombin time, normally 11 to 14 seconds, indicates the amount of prothrombin available for clotting of the blood. The prothrombin is lowered when anticoagulant drugs, such as heparin, Coumadin (warfarin) and Dicumarol (bishydroxycoumarin) are given to patients to reduce the clotting tendency of the blood. Myocardial infarction, thromboembolism and vascular thromboses are frequently treated with anticoagulants. A daily test is done to determine how much of the anticoagulant should be given. The therapeutic range is between 10 and 30 per cent of normal activity.

BLOOD SUGAR

The diabetic patient is subject to myocardial infarction as a result of advanced atherosclerosis. The blood sugar, normally 70 to 120 mg./ml. (fasting), may be elevated during the attack. Occasionally an acute myocardial infarct may precipitate diabetes in a latent diabetic.

BLOOD-UREA NITROGEN

This test is used to evaluate kidney function. The blood-urea nitrogen will be elevated if cardiac output is reduced. Normal range is 10 to 20 mg. per 100 ml. of blood.

SERUM CHOLESTEROL

Cholesterol is important in body metabolism. In atherosclerosis, deposits of cholesterol and other lipids are found in the connective tissue of the arterial walls. The increased cholesterol level is probably due to faulty lipid metabolism. Normal range is 150 to 290 mg. per 100 ml. of blood.

SODIUM

Sodium is the chief cation of the blood and extracellular fluid. It is associated with bicarbonate to regulate the acid-base balance in the blood, and with potassium to maintain normal heart action. Sodium concentration is frequently diminished in patients with congestive heart failure as a result of a low sodium intake together with fluid retention, treatment with diuretics, and impaired renal function. Normal range is 135 to 145 mEq. per liter of serum.

POTASSIUM

Potassium is the principal cation of intracellular fluid with a normal concentration of 3.5 to 5 mEq. per liter of serum. It is chiefly concerned with cellular osmosis and muscle activity. A marked decrease in potassium may cause cardiac arrhythmia.

CHLORIDES

Chlorides constitute the chief anion of the extracellular fluid, with a normal concentration of 95 to 105 mEq. per liter of serum. Its chief function is to control osmotic pressure. An increase is noted in heart failure with kidney impairment. This is due to the inability of the kidneys to properly eliminate sodium and chloride.

CO_2 COMBINING POWER

This test measures the pH level of the blood. Normal concentration is 24 to 32 mEq. per liter of serum, and indicates the amount of base bicarbonate available to combine with cations. An increase in CO_2 combining power usually indicates metabolic alkalosis and respiratory acidosis, while a decrease indicates metabolic acidosis and respiratory alkalosis.

Serum Enzyme Tests

Enzymes are complex protein substances found in the serum and tissues. Transaminases are enzymes found in the heart, liver, muscle, kidneys and pancreas. Injury to one of these organs releases the transaminase from the damaged cell into the serum. Following infarction there is a transient increase according to the extent of the damage.

SERUM GLUTAMIC OXALOACETIC TRANSAMINASE

The normal SGOT range is 8 to 40 units. After an acute myocardial infarction the level rises 3 times its normal level and and may rise as high as 500 to 600 units in 12 to 48 hours. It usually returns to normal within 4 to 7 days.

SERUM GLUTAMIC PYRUVIC TRANSAMINASE

The normal SGPT range is 5 to 35 units. It is used mainly in the diagnosis of hepatitis. However, the SGPT can indicate whether a rise in the SGOT is due to myocardial damage or heart failure. In heart failure the SGPT is higher than the SGOT.

SERUM LACTIC DEHYDROGENASE

The normal SLDH range is 100 to 350 units. This test is used chiefly as an aid in the diagnosis of myocardial infarction. Its level rises 2 to 10 times its normal 12 to 24 hours after infarction and persists for 10 to 12 days. Electrophoretic analysis indicates that of the 5 isoenzymes of SLDH it is the fifth isoenzyme that accounts for most of the elevation.

SERUM CREATINE PHOSPHOKINASE

The normal SCPK range is 0 to 4 units. It is found in skeletal muscle and heart muscle. In acute myocardial infarction its level rises 6 hours after infarction to 5 times its normal within 24 hours. It usually returns to normal within 72 hours.

SERUM ALPHA-HYDROXYBUTYRATE DEHYDROGENASE

The normal SHBD rate is 50 to 150 units. This test is used chiefly to confirm the diagnosis of myocardial infarction. Its level rises within 12 hours after infarction and persists for 1 to 3 weeks.

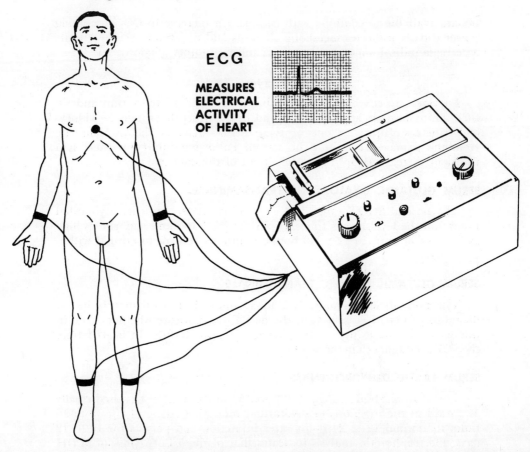

ECG

MEASURES
ELECTRICAL
ACTIVITY
OF HEART

FIG. 2–1. Placement of standard leads.

THE ELECTROCARDIOGRAM

The electrocardiogram is a graphic representation of changes in the electrical potential of the heart. A small amount of electrical energy is generated by the heart during each cardiac cycle. Each normal cardiac cell maintains an electrical potential. At rest the potential is negative, but immediately following contraction it becomes positive. The impulses which precede contraction arise in the conduction system of the heart. By applying electrodes to various positions on the body and connecting these electrodes to the electrocardiograph machine, the electrical energy is picked up, amplified and recorded on moving graph paper.

The bipolar standard leads shown in Figure 2–1 were selected in 1903 by Einthoven, who labeled the changes in potential as the P, QRS and T waves. The bipolar leads record the difference in potential of two points on the frontal plane of the body.

Bipolar standard leads are attached in the following manner:

LEAD	POSITIVE CONNECTION	NEGATIVE CONNECTION
I	Left arm	Right arm
II	Left leg	Right arm
III	Left leg	Left arm

The precordial, or chest leads, are unipolar and demonstrate differences of potential between any one of eight positions on the chest and one extremity.

The precordial leads are attached in the following positions:

V_1 4th intercostal space at the right sternal border

V_2 4th intercostal space at the left sternal border

V_3 Between the 4th and 5th intercostal spaces equidistant between V_2 and V_4

V_4 5th intercostal space in the left midclavicular line

V_5 5th intercostal space in the left anterior axillary line

V_6 5th intercostal space in the left midaxillary line

V_7 5th intercostal space in the left posterior axillary line

V_8 5th intercostal space at the left posterior scapular line

Unipolar (augmented) limb leads register the electric variations at one point. Due to their distance from the heart, these leads produce small deflections in the ECG. The electrocardiographic machine slightly augments these leads, hence they are called aVR, aVL and aVF. The "a" means that it is augmented, the V signifies Vector, or unipolar, lead and the R, L, F refer to the specific extremity. These leads are attached in the following positions:

aVR   Right arm

aVL   Left arm

aVF   Left leg

Excitation of cardiac muscle is accomplished by two processes:

1. Spontaneous development of an impulse in the automatic pacemaker cell
2. Conduction of this impulse from fiber to fiber throughout the heart musculature

Generally, it may be said that cardiac arrhythmias result from disturbances in impulse formation, disturbances in conduction of the impulse, or disturbances in both. To recognize or identify abnormal

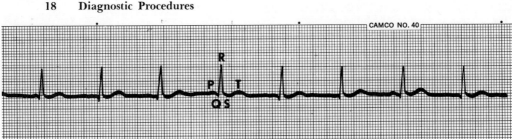

FIG. 2–2. Normal electrocardiogram.

rhythms on the ECG tracing, the nurse should have a thorough understanding of the normal heart cycle and the time relationships of the events which occur.

The normal cardiac cycle shown in Figure 2–2 shows a heart rate of 68, P-R interval of 0.16 second, and QRS complex of 0.08 second.

The ECG paper consists of small squares outlined by a dark line every fifth square. Each small square is 0.1 mm. apart and represents a potential of 0.1 millivolt, with a time interval of 0.04 second. The P, QRS and T waves are graphed on the paper in terms of:

1. **Polarity.** Positive voltage gives an upward deflection; negative voltage gives a downward deflection. Isoelectric voltage, indicating that the electrodes have equal potential, is recorded as zero, or a straight line.
2. **Magnitude.** The wave is measured by its relation to the horizontal lines.
3. **Duration.** The wave is measured by its relation to the vertical lines.

DEFINITION OF EVENTS

1. **Depolarization.** Loss of electrical charge.
2. **Repolarization.** Build-up of electrical charge.
3. **Polarized.** Resting phase.
4. **P wave.** A positive deflection produced by the spread of electrical energy throughout the atria (depolarization).
5. **Q wave.** First negative deflection in the QRS complex.
6. **R wave.** First positive deflection in the QRS complex.
7. **S wave.** Negative deflection following the R wave.
8. **QRS complex.** Produced by the spread of electrical energy throughout the ventricles (depolarization).
9. **T wave.** A positive deflection, corresponding to the resting phase of the ventricles.
10. **U wave.** Positive deflection following the T wave.
11. **Refractory.** Resistance of cardiac tissue to restimulation during the peak of fast action potential.

TIMING EVENTS

All electrocardiograms are standardized so that 5 large squares of the graph paper move under the writing stylus each second. Each large square represents 0.2 second at normal paper speed through the machine. In one minute, 300 large squares go by the stylus. One method used to calculate the heart rate is to count the number of 0.2-second intervals between the peaks of the two R waves and divide into 300. Thus two R waves separated by 4½ 0.2-second squares would represent 68 beats per minute.

1. **P-R interval.** The time interval from the beginning of atrial depolarization to the beginning of ventricular depolarization, and measured from the start of the P wave to the beginning of the R wave. The normal duration is from 0.12 to 0.20 second.
2. **QRS complex.** Measured from the start of the Q wave to the end of the S wave. The normal duration is from 0.05 to 0.1 second.
3. **S-T segment.** Lies between the QRS complex and the T wave. The normal duration is from 0.14 to 0.16 second.
4. **Q-T interval.** Measured from the start of the QRS complex to the end of the T wave. The normal duration is less than 0.43 second.
5. **P-P interval.** Time between two consecutive P waves.

The electrocardiogram is valuable in the diagnosis of many types of heart disease, but its major use is in the diagnosis of coronary heart disease and in identifying cardiac arrhythmias.

REFERENCES AND BIBLIOGRAPHY

Bernreiter, M.: Electrocardiography. ed. 2. Philadelphia, J. B. Lippincott, 1963.

Collins, R. D.: Illustrated Manual of Laboratory Diagnosis. Philadelphia, J. B. Lippincott, 1968.

French, R.: Nurse's Guide to Diagnostic Procedures. ed. 2. pp. 51-146. New York, McGraw-Hill, 1967.

Goldman, M. J.: Principles of Clinical Electrocardiography. pp. 25-30, 45-61, 328-329. Los Altos, California, Lange Medical Publications, 1967.

Goodall, R.: Clinical Interpretation of Laboratory Tests. ed. 5. pp. 29-82, 97-137, 315-316. Philadelphia, F. A. Davis, 1965.

Wood, P.: Diseases of the Heart and Circulation. ed. 3. Philadelphia, J. B. Lippincott, 1968.

3 THE DEVELOPMENT OF CORONARY ARTERY DISEASE

Heart disease continues to be the leading cause of death in the United States.[1] Poor living habits are predisposing millions of Americans to coronary artery disease. Preventive measures, initiated early in life, present the best opportunity of delaying or retarding coronary heart disease.

Coronary artery disease may be defined as an occlusion of the coronary arteries which interferes with the blood supply to the cardiac muscle, resulting in myocardial ischemia. Atherosclerosis is the most common disease of the coronary arteries. Fatty granulomatous lesions (atheromas) develop in the inner walls of the artery and interfere with the circulation of blood by narrowing the lumen of the artery. Intramural hemorrhage may occur, resulting in occlusion. Figure 3–1 demonstrates the gradual deterioration of a diseased artery.

ETIOLOGY

Although the cause of coronary artery disease is unknown, certain factors increase the incidence of atherosclerosis: genetic factors, dietary habits, hypertension, diabetes mellitus, stress, smoking, sex and lack of exercise. Some of these factors may play interrelated roles in the rate of development of atherosclerosis, while others may precipitate an acute cardiac event.

Heredity and environment influence the structural components of the arterial system where atheromas develop. A family history of coronary artery disease may be due to a tendency to atherosclerosis resulting from any combination of the risk factors.

Foods high in saturated fat, cholesterol and calories raise the blood cholesterol, contributing to the development of atherosclerosis.

---

[1] What Are the Pay-Offs From Our Federal Health Programs? A Progress Report on the Johnson Administration—1963 to 1968. p. 19. New York, National Health Education Committee, 1968.

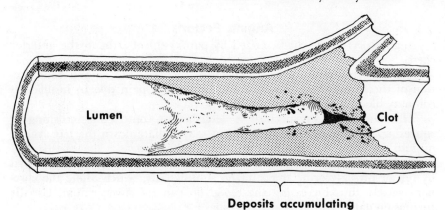

Fig. 3–1. Occluded coronary artery.

The increased pressure in the arterial wall which exists with hypertension increases the frequency of atherosclerosis.

Coronary artery disease is seen frequently in patients who have a fat or sugar metabolic disorder, or who have a familial history of diabetes mellitus. Uncontrolled diabetes increases the blood cholesterol level. Vascular changes in the lower extremities, eyes and kidneys are common. Circulatory disorders are, in many instances, the immediate cause of the diabetic's death.

Constant environmental stress strains the individual's adjustment processes. If the stress level is consistently above his ability to cope with it, consequent disturbances in metabolism contribute to an increase of cholesterol.

Cigarette smoking is an added risk for people who are susceptible to coronary disease. Nicotine, a toxic substance, raises the blood pressure, makes the heart beat faster, acts as a vasoconstrictor and increases the heart's need for oxygen.

Men suffer more complications of atherosclerosis than do women of the same age before menopause. In women, estrogen secretion acts as a protective mechanism. After age 40, women show a slow but constant rise in coronary disease up to age 70.

Obesity contributes to exertional dyspnea and dependent edema, and also elevates the blood pressure. Lack of physical exercise predisposes one to obesity. Daily exercise stimulates the circulation, aids muscle tone and helps to stabilize weight.

EFFECTS OF CORONARY ARTERY DISEASE

Disease of the inner walls of the coronary arteries results in obstruction of blood flow to the heart. This event leads to a number of different types of clinical syndromes, caused by myocardial ischemia.

Angina Pectoris

Angina pectoris is characterized by paroxysms of pain in the anterior chest.

Any activity, stress, or emotion which increases the oxygen consumption of the myocardium may precipitate anginal pain due to insufficient coronary blood flow and myocardial hypoxia.

The pain of angina pectoris is described as constricting, crushing or squeezing. Usually it is substernal, but may radiate down the left arm or up into the neck. Dyspnea may accompany the pain.

In classical angina, the pain lasts for 5 minutes or less, and is relieved by rest or nitroglycerin tablets, taken sublingually, which dilate the coronary vessels, thus increasing the blood flow to the myocardium. Usually there is no damage to myocardial tissue.

Coronary Insufficiency

Coronary insufficiency refers to an attack in which the cardiac pain is more prolonged than the pain of angina pectoris and may last from 15 minutes to half an hour.

This event is due to inadequate circulation resulting from atherosclerosis. Undue stress, emotional crisis or physical strain may be the precipitating factor causing a temporary constriction of the coronary artery.

Syncope sometimes accompanies the pain, and a drop in blood pressure is not unusual. The pain of insufficiency is less easily relieved by rest or nitroglycerin tablets, but may finally be relieved by sedation.

Coronary Thrombosis

Coronary thrombosis occurs when a clot forms in the narrowed and roughened part of the artery, blocking the lumen. Intimal capillaries are prone to rupture. Such occlusion resulting from clot formation may develop either suddenly or gradually. If collateral circulation is sufficient to supply the myocardium, occlusion may occur without infarction.

The symptoms are similar to those of myocardial infarction. The individual complains of persistent, severe precordial pain. Blood pressure may drop suddenly or gradually, accompanied by signs of shock such as a rapid, irregular pulse, pallor, cold sweat, apprehension and restlessness. Nausea and vomiting are not unusual, and the individual may attribute this as well as his pain to an attack of indigestion.

The patient admitted with a coronary thrombosis requires intensive care and should be monitored for signs of an impending infarction.

Myocardial Infarction

Myocardial infarction, a destruction of heart muscle due to ischemia, is a major disaster facing the patient with coronary artery disease. The pain of myocardial infarction varies from an uncomfortable sense of pressure in the chest, gradually reaching a peak intensity of excruciating agony. Similar to the pain of angina pectoris, it may radiate to the neck, shoulders and upper extremities.

SYMPTOMS

The individual may describe the intense substernal pain as sharp, stabbing, crushing, constant or oppressive. It may occur while the individual is sleeping or resting, but may be induced by exertion and stress.

With the increasing severity of the pain as well as its persistence, the individual becomes extremely restless and apprehensive. He may become panicky and walk about clutching his chest, unable to breathe properly.

Shock may be the outstanding characteristic in those individuals relatively free from pain. A sudden reduction in cardiac output due to the damaged myocardium may cause the individual to feel weak, and he may collapse. His blood pressure drops and his pulse is rapid and weak, accompanied by dyspnea. His skin is cold and clammy and he usually exhibits an ashen gray cyanosis. He may display anxiety, or his countenance may appear dazed and listless.

In the majority of patients with myocardial infarction, pain is the predominant symptom. Several hours after onset, the blood pressure may fall to shock levels. This results from decreased cardiac output, which is responsible for peripheral vasoconstriction and tachycardia. The pulse pressure decreases and the pulse becomes thready. The patient feels weak and dyspneic. Nausea and vomiting may occur.

A rise in temperature is noted at the end of the first day and persists for about a week. It returns to normal with the development of collateral circulation and tissue repair.

LABORATORY FINDINGS IN MYOCARDIAL INFARCTION

Leukocytosis and an increased sedimentation rate appear within 48 hours. Serum enzyme studies show an increase in serum glutamic oxalo-acetic transaminase activity within 12 to 48 hours and lasting 4 to 7 days. Serum lactic dehydrogenase elevation occurs 6 to 12 hours after infarction and returns to normal within 10 to 12 days. Serum creatine phosphokinase is elevated 6 to 12 hours after infarction and returns to normal within 72 hours.

Electrocardiograph changes following infarction are determined by the location of the infarct and the extent of damage to the muscle cells.

TREATMENT AND NURSING RESPONSIBILITIES

Medical treatment and nursing care are designed to:

1. Relieve pain
2. Alleviate shock

3. Provide rest for the injured heart
4. Prevent complications
5. Achieve maximum rehabilitation

The moment the patient enters the coronary care unit the nurse makes a rapid assessment of his physical and emotional status. She then establishes priorities of care, and acts promptly to implement them. Patients in acute distress usually have at least one complicating factor. If such an emergency exists, the nurse initiates the treatment program for the complication.

Medication is given to relieve pain. With the relief of pain, apprehension will be lessened and the patient may be able to rest.

If the patient is in shock, treatment must be started immediately if death is to be prevented. The nurse should:

1. Start oxygen immediately to combat tissue hypoxia.
2. Start intravenous glucose with a vasopressor to maintain systolic pressure at 100.
3. Take apical-radial pulse to determine the pulse deficit.
4. Record blood pressure and pulse rate frequently.
5. Be alert for the development of arrhythmias.

As soon as possible after admission, electrodes should be placed on the patient and a rhythm strip obtained. At this time the nurse should explain the monitoring concept to the patient, take and record T.P.R. (temperature, pulse, respiration), blood pressure and apical-radial pulse. Throughout these critical moments of caring for the patient, the nurse must be sensitive to the overwhelming psychological as well as physical impact of the emergency. What she does and says should add to the patient's confidence and comfort.

NURSING CARE SUBSEQUENT TO ADMISSION

1. Continuously assess the patient's cardiac status.
2. Be alert to the heart rhythm on the oscilloscope; be able to distinguish all significant arrhythmias at their onset, and notify the physician if indicated.
3. Assess other sources of difficulty, such as signs and symptoms of congestive heart failure, pulmonary embolism and shock.
4. Note effect of medications.
5. Maintain hygiene and physical comfort, exercising discretion about such needs as baths and linen changes.
6. View the patient as a complete individual and do not confine observations of him to the monitor.
7. Identify and plan to meet his other needs.

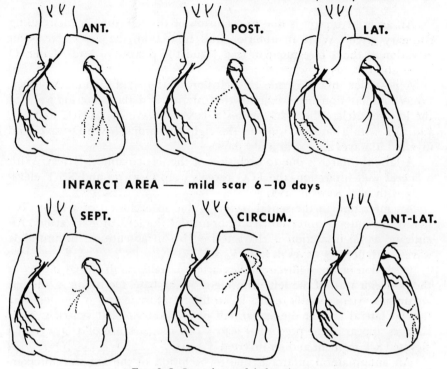

FIG. 3–2. Locations of infarction.

Location of Infarctions

In most instances the site of an infarction can be anatomically located by observing the progressive changes in the various ECG leads. The dead zone of a myocardial infarction is electrically inert; hence, during the early period of ventricular depolarization, the electrical forces generated in the opposite region of the heart dominate the electrical field.

Abnormalities resulting from acute myocardial infarction are:

1. An abnormal negative Q wave
2. A deformity in the RS-T segment elevated above the isoelectric line in leads I or III
3. Depression of the S-T segment
4. The inversion of T waves after several weeks, and their abnormal symmetry

However, myocardial infarction may be present without significant changes in the ECG.

The locations of the infarctions are illustrated by the dotted lines in each of the drawings in Figure 3–2.

An **anterior** infarct is due to occlusion of the left anterior descending coronary artery. With an anterior wall infarction, the ECG reveals an elevation of the S-T segment in lead I and the precordial leads. Later, Q waves and inverted T waves appear.

A **posterior** infarct is due to occlusion of the right circumflex artery. Posterior infarction involves both the inferior and the posterior walls of the left ventricle. The ECG reveals a large Q wave in leads II and III, and aVF with a large R wave in the right precordial leads. Q waves and inverted T waves appear in a few days.

A **lateral** infarct is due to occlusion of the left circumflex artery. With a lateral wall infarction, the ECG reveals deep Q waves and RS-T elevations with a T wave in aVL.

An infarction in the **septal** region is due to occlusion of a right division of the anterior interventricular branch of the left coronary artery. An anterior septal infarction is characterized by an absence of the initial R waves, with deep Q waves in leads V_2 and V_3.

Occlusion of the right **circumflex** artery usually results in an infarct of the posterior wall of the left ventricle near the base. Occlusion of the left circumflex artery usually results in an infarct of some area of the left ventricular lateral wall or the apical half of the posterior left ventricle. ECG changes appear in the precordial lead V_6 by the presence of a Q wave, an elevated S-T segment and an inverted T wave.

An **anterolateral** infarct is due to occlusion of the anterior interventricular branch of the left coronary artery. In anterolateral infarction the ECG reveals an R wave in the right precordial leads V_1 and V_2 which disappears in the more lateral leads. A Q wave with a Q-S or Q-R complex appears in V_4, V_5 or V_6.

Patterns of Myocardial Damage

ISCHEMIA

When the flow to a coronary artery is cut off, the first ECG change is T wave inversion, as shown in Figure 3–3. Due to loss of cell membrane integrity, polarization cannot occur, resulting in changes in the repolarization phase of the P-QRS-T cycle. If the ischemia becomes more severe,

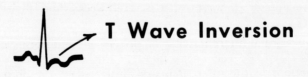 T Wave Inversion

Figure 3–3

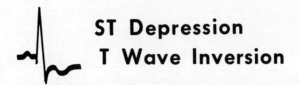

ST Depression
T Wave Inversion

FIGURE 3–4

S-T depression also occurs, as shown in Figure 3–4. These changes are reversible.

INJURY

Injured heart muscle stays depolarized. The "current of injury" is the current which flows from the normally polarized area to the pathologically depolarized area. This results in S-T segment elevation and continued T

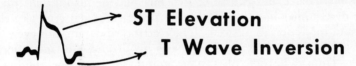

ST Elevation
T Wave Inversion

FIGURE 3–5

wave inversion, as indicated in Figure 3–5. This change is still reversible, and can be seen in impending infarction.

INFARCTION

The injury to the myocardium is now irreversible—death has occurred through the muscle wall. Dead tissue has no electrical activity. An electrode placed over the infarcted area will show a pathological Q wave, as

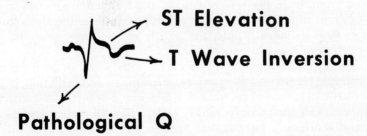

ST Elevation
T Wave Inversion

Pathological Q

FIGURE 3–6

shown in Figure 3–6, because the electrical activity of the opposite side of the heart is being recorded and the depolarization wave is moving away

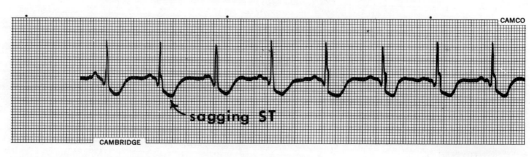

FIG. 3–7. Ischemia.

from the electrode. As recovery occurs, the injury pattern (S-T elevation and T inversion) will disappear, but the pathological Q will remain, though it may become smaller.

The occurrence and course of ischemia and/or myocardial infarction can be determined in the ECG by the presence of patterns of ischemia, injury and infarction in all leads. The electrocardiogram, however, is only one diagnostic tool. The physician bases his diagnosis of infarction on a complete clinical history, physical examination, laboratory findings and clinical judgment.

There is a broad spectrum of "normal" distribution of the coronary arteries. There is also a wide variation in degree of collateral circulation. The occlusion of a specific site may be relatively benign in one person, while life threatening to another in whose heart there is little collateral circulation, resulting in damage to a larger area of the heart, or whose circulation to a vital zone such as the conduction system depends upon the occluded vessel for nutrition.

The common opinion is that the S-A node is provided by the right coronary artery in 55 per cent of people, and by the left circumflex artery in 45 per cent of people. The A-V node is provided by the right coronary artery in 90 per cent of people, and by the left coronary artery in 10 per cent of people.

The arrhythmias most often associated with posterior wall infarction are premature ventricular contractions, atrial flutter or fibrillation, left bundle branch block, partial or total A-V block and ventricular tachycardia.

Anterior wall infarction is mostly associated with right bundle branch block and ventricular tachycardia. Anteroseptal infarction is mostly associated with right bundle branch block.

Figure 3–7 presents the sagging S-T segment of ischemia. No arrhythmia is present.

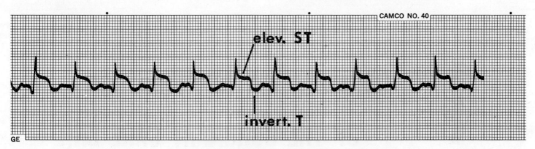

Fig. 3–8. Acute injury pattern.

Figure 3–8 presents the acute injury pattern. Present are S-T segment elevation, inverted T wave and pathological Q. No arrhythmia is present.

REFERENCES AND BIBLIOGRAPHY

Bernreiter, M.: Electrocardiography. ed. 2. Philadelphia, J. B. Lippincott, 1963.

Braun, H. A., and Diettert, G. A.: Coronary Care Unit Nursing. ed. 3. Missoula, Montana, Western Montana Clinic Foundation, 1968.

Brunner, L. S., Emerson, C. P., Ferguson, L. K., and Suddarth, D. S.: Textbook of Medical-Surgical Nursing. ed. 2. pp. 359-392. Philadelphia, J. B. Lippincott, 1970.

Friedberg, C. K.: Diseases of the Heart. ed. 3. pp. 219-242, 284-304, 443-474, 483-575, 583-628, 643-693, 676-678, 706-763, 770-791, 866-922. Philadelphia, W. B. Saunders, 1966.

Guyton, A. C.: Textbook of Medical Physiology. ed. 3. pp. 179-194, 233-243, 301-310, 312-320, 371-382. Philadelphia, W. B. Saunders, 1966.

Hurst, J. W., and Logue, R. R.: The Heart. pp. 224-234, 239-282, 285-341, 350-362. New York, McGraw-Hill, 1966.

MacBryde, C. M.: Signs and Symptoms.

ed. 4. pp. 262-308, 225. Philadelphia, J. B. Lippincott, 1964.

Meltzer, L. E., et al: Intensive Coronary Care—A Manual for Nurses. CCU Fund, Philadelphia Presbyterian Hospital, 1965.

Metheny, N. M., and Snively, W. D.: Nurses' Handbook of Fluid Balance. pp. 195-211. Philadelphia, J. B. Lippincott, 1967.

Shafer, K. N., Sawyer, J. R., McClusky, A.M., and Beck, E. L.: Medical-Surgical Nursing. ed. 4. pp. 317-346, 358-361. St. Louis, C. V. Mosby, 1967.

Smith, D. W., and Gips, C. D.: Care of the Adult Patient. ed. 2. pp. 529-580, 627-637. Philadelphia, J. B. Lippincott, 1966.

What Are the Pay-Offs From Our Federal Health Programs? A Progress Report on the Johnson Administration—1963-1968. p. 19. New York, National Health Education Committee, 1968.

Wood, P.: Diseases of the Heart and Circulation. ed. 3. Philadelphia, J. B. Lippincott, 1968.

4 ORGANIZATION AND FUNCTION OF THE CORONARY CARE UNIT

An increasing knowledge of coronary artery disease has not altered the fact that it is still the nation's leading health problem. While national efforts continue to research the causative factors, hospitals must provide the equipment and staff necessary to give competent, intensive coronary care.

The primary purpose of the coronary care unit is to reduce the high mortality associated with the disease by terminating the major arrhythmias and by giving successful resuscitation. To meet this objective, a specially designed unit within the hospital must be equipped and staffed to provide an effective team of skilled medical and nursing personnel.

After the decision to establish a coronary care unit has been made, the hospital must concern itself with policies regarding medical and nursing responsibilities. The following discussion of policies and organization gives a general picture of the organization of a coronary care unit. The nurse practicing in this area needs a clear understanding of how she fits into the overall system of patient care, and what her responsibilities are. The nursing staff is responsible for determining standards of nursing care in the coronary care unit.

ORGANIZATION

The department of cardiology supervises and guides ongoing care and techniques of treatment. Members serve on a rotating basis and are responsible during their tour of duty for daily review of the unit activities. They review case management with the house staff. By admitting their patients to the unit, physicians agree that emergency measures may be instituted by the medical or nursing staff in attendance during emergencies such as arrhythmias. Procedures are designed to anticipate, detect and aggressively treat the complications of coronary disease such as arrhythmias, cardio-genic shock, cardiac arrest and cardiac decompensation.

All patients are under the care of the assigned cardiologist.

If the concept of the coronary care unit is to be achieved, nurses working in the unit must be prepared and authorized to:

1. Start and maintain oxygen therapy.
2. Start rotating tourniquet machines or manual tourniquet rotation in acute pulmonary edema.
3. Attach electrodes and maintain constant monitoring.
4. Initiate closed chest massage manually or utilize an automatic massage machine.
5. Use equipment to assist respirations.
6. Use and regulate the external pacemaker in cardiac arrest.
7. Initiate cardiac defibrillation in cardiac standstill.
8. Begin intravenous medications, including the use of Medi-Cut or Rochester needle with intracatheter.
9. Draw blood for blood chemistry determinations when necessary.

CRITERIA FOR ADMISSION

Patients, either male or female, with a diagnosis of definite or suspected acute myocardial infarction, as well as patients with cardiac arrhythmias in need of the supervision, care and monitoring facilities of the unit are admitted.

MECHANISM OF ADMISSION

Requests for admission to the coronary care unit are made by the attending physician through the nurse in charge of the unit.

1. If a bed is available, the nurse in charge notifies the admitting office.
2. If a bed is not available, the medical resident must decide whether or not one of the patients in the unit may be transferred out.

DISCHARGE

1. The decision to discharge a patient from the unit is made by the attending physician and, in case of prolonged stay, the final decision as to occupancy of a bed in the unit is made by the chief cardiologist.
2. The patient with a myocardial infarction is usually transferred out of the unit when he has been free of complications for 3 days.

GENERAL POLICIES

VISITORS

Visiting is limited to one visitor at a time. The time and length of the visit is determined by the nurse in charge and depends on the condition of the patient and the condition of the unit in general.

CORONARY CARE UNIT
DOCTOR'S ORDER SHEET

A. Coronary intensive care unit nurses are permitted to do the following on this patient:

1. Start and maintain oxygen therapy at their discretion.

2. Begin intravenous infusions with 5% D/W and add intravenous medications on physician's written or oral order. They may use Medi-Cut or Rochester needle with intracatheter.

3. Draw blood for blood chemistry determinations.

4. Start rotating tourniquets or rotating tourniquet machine in acute pulmonary edema.

5. Attach electrodes and maintain constant monitoring.

6. Perform closed chest massage manually or utilize automatic massage machine.

7. Use equipment to assist respiration including a manual breathing bag and/or airway.

8. Use and regulate the external pacemaker if cardiac arrest occurs.

9. In "Cardiac Standstill" (no cardiac output), the first qualified person to arrive institutes therapy. This includes nursing personnel.

B. Permission is granted to members of the coronary care committee to review the medical record of _____.
                                                 (Patient's Name)

Signed: _____M.D.

Date: _____

FIGURE 4–1

When not actually visiting a patient, visitors are asked to use a special waiting room adjacent to the unit.

RADIO AND TELEVISION

Radios and televisions are allowed only by order of the physician.

SMOKING

Smoking is not permitted by anyone.

RECORDS

1. **Consent for Defibrillation.** The patient or his next of kin is asked to sign the regular hospital form, Consent for Operation or Treatment.
2. **Electrocardiogram.** A daily ECG report is attached to the patient's permanent record.
3. **Doctor's Order Sheet, Coronary Care Unit.** The attending physician's signature authorizes the coronary care unit nurses to function within the limits of hospital policy. (See Fig. 4–1 for sample of doctor's order sheet.)

REPORTS

1. A report on all patients is prepared by the charge nurse on each shift.
2. A report on all patients is made by the supervisor and/or charge nurse every morning and sent to the director of nursing service who in turn sends it to the director of the hospital.

CENSUS BOOK

For purposes of research, a record of each patient admitted to the coronary care unit is kept in the census book and includes: date, bed number, time of admission, diagnosis, age, attending physician, date and time of discharge and course of illness.

CARDIAC ARREST BOOK

A record of each patient treated by the cardiac arrest team is kept and includes: date, room, name of patient, diagnosis, age, attending physician and course of illness.

CHARTING

The patient's chart includes a special check list which the nurse completes when the patient is admitted. The check list, an example of which is shown in Figure 4–2, ensures a complete nursing assessment of each patient on admission.

CORONARY CARE UNIT

BEDSIDE ADMISSION NOTES

CHARGE PLATE

DATE: _____

TIME: _____

CHAIR: _____ AMBULATORY: _____ STRETCHER: _____

TRANSFER IN FROM: _____

BLOOD PRESSURE RT. ARM: _____ LEFT ARM: _____

PULSE APICAL: _____ RADIAL: _____ DEFICIT: _____

TEMPERATURE ORAL: _____ AXILLARY: _____

RESPIRATION DYSPNEA: _____ RALES: _____

    COUGH: _____ SPUTUM: _____ HEMOPTYSIS: _____

    WHEEZING: _____ CHEYNE-STOKES: _____

    KUSSMAUL: _____ APNEA: _____

BREATH ODOR ACETONE: _____ ALCOHOL: _____

PAIN TIME OF ONSET: _____ LOCATION: _____

    SEVERITY: _____ DURATION: _____

    HOW RELIEVED: _____ HOW AGGRAVATED: _____

DIAPHORESIS: _____ CYANOSIS: _____ PALLOR: _____

    FLUSHING: _____ EDEMA: _____ COLD EXTREMITIES: _____

    DISTENTION OF NECK VEINS: _____

RECENT URINE OUTPUT: _____ URINE SPECIMEN OBTAINED: _____

OXYGEN: _____

EMOTIONAL STATE: _____

STATE OF CONSCIOUSNESS: _____

MONITOR APPLIED: _____ MONITOR EXPLAINED: _____

RHYTHM STRIP RUN: _____

DESCRIPTION OF RHYTHM STRIP: _____

ECG DONE: _____ RESIDENT NOTIFIED: _____

PHYSICIAN NOTIFIED: _____

MEDICAL HISTORY

    HEART DISEASE: _____ PREVIOUS CORONARY: _____

    ANGINA: _____ DIABETES: _____ ASTHMA: _____

    EMPHYSEMA: _____ ALLERGIES: _____ OTHER: _____

MEDICATION HISTORY

    NITROGLYCERIN: _____ DIURETICS: _____

    DIGITALIS: _____ QUINIDINE: _____

    ANTICOAGULANTS: _____ ANTICONVULSANTS: _____

    INSULIN: _____ OTHER: _____

CLOTHES AND VALUABLES CARED FOR BY: _____

RELATIVES INSTRUCTED AND GIVEN CCU PAMPHLET: _____

OTHER PERTINENT INFORMATION:

HEIGHT: _____ WEIGHT: _____

FIGURE 4–2

NURSES NOTES	COR. I. - C.C.U. BROWN, CHARLES 201000 M45 3456127 M.S. BENTLEY -H-

DATE	MEDICATION AND TREATMENTS	HOUR	TIME	OBSERVATIONS	DOCTOR'S VISITS
10/4/69			11 AM	45 YEAR OLD MAN	
				BROUGHT TO EMERGENCY	
				ROOM BY POLICE SCOUT	
				CAR, OFFICER J. WALTERS,	
				BADGE #7719.	
	TEMP 97 (ORAL)			PATIENT IS ACCOMPANIED	
	B.P. RIGHT ARM 100/80			BY WIFE.	
	LEFT ARM 96/88			COMPLAINS OF SEVERE	
	A/R 130/120			SUB-STERNAL PAIN OF	
	NASAL OXYGEN 6 4/m	11:05		2 HOURS DURATION, WHICH	
	EGG AND C.B.C. DONE	11:15		PATIENT DESCRIBES AS	
				"INDIGESTION," UNRELIEVED	
				BY ALKALIES. NO	
				RADIATION OF PAIN. SKIN	
				COOL AND CLAMMY, VERY	
				SLIGHT DYSPNEA, COLOR	
				PALE.	
				EXAM BY	DR. JONES
				DR. BENTLEY NOTIFIED	
	MORPHINE S. gr. 1/6 I.V.	11 05/AM			
			11:30	TRANSFERRED TO CORONARY	
				CARE UNIT BY BED LITTER	
				WITH PORTABLE OXYGEN.	
				Elizabeth Allen R.N.	
	BP RIGHT ARM 96/78		11:35 AM	ADMITTED TO C.C.U. AND	
	LEFT ARM 94/76			CLOTHING LISTED BY M. Davis R.N.	
	TEMP 97 RESP. 24			PATIENT STATES PAIN HAS	
	A/R 116/116			BEEN RELIEVED BY DRUG IN	
	MONITOR APPLIED + EXPLAINED			E.R SINUS TACHYCARDIA RATE	
	ADMISSION STRIP RUN			116-120 RARE PVC. P-R 0.2	
	NASAL OXYGEN CONT'D.		11:40 AM	SEEN BY DR. BENTLEY	
	1000cc 5% %/w STARTED		11:45 AM	PATIENT STATES HIS	
	WITH MED. INTRACATH			PAIN IS COMPLETELY	
	AS KEEP-OPEN I.V. IN LEFT ARM			GONE.	

NURSES NOTES

Fig. 4–3. Chart for a 24-hour period, including 8-hour summary statements.

EIGHT-HOUR SUMMARY CHARTING

End-of-shift charting includes:

1. Description of end-of-shift rhythm strip
   a. Rate—apical/radial, pulse deficit if any

DATE	MEDICATION AND TREATMENTS	HOUR	TIME	OBSERVATIONS	DOCTOR'S VISITS
10/4/69	BLOOD FOR ENZYMES AND SED. RATE	11:40	11:45	SKIN NOW DRY AND RESP. EASY COLOR FAIR.	
	HEIGHT 6'			QUITE TALKATIVE AND SEEMS	
	WEIGHT 198 #			NERVOUS. STATES THIS IS	
				HIS FIRST EPISODE OF	
	BP. 110/80	11:45		CHEST PAIN, WHICH HE IS	
				SURE IS INDIGESTION.	
				CANNOT SEE WHY HE HAS	
				BEEN PLACED IN A "HEART	
				WARD." PREVENTIVE ASPECT	
				OF C.C.U. EXPLAINED.	
				PATIENT IS A SELF-EMPLOYED	
				BUSINESSMAN, WITH MUCH	
				TENSION ASSOCIATED WITH	
	NO KNOWN ALLERGIES			WORK. NO PAST MEDICAL	
				HISTORY, ESPECIALLY DIABETES	
				OR CARDIAC.	
				DENIES ANY CALF PAIN.	
				NO EDEMA OF LOWER EXTREMITIES.	
	BP. 100/80	12:00	12:00	PATIENT CONTINUES TO	
				PROTEST HIS ADMISSION TO	
				THIS UNIT.	
				ADMITS TO HAVING SEVERAL	
				MILD EPISODES OF "INDIGESTION."	
				THE PAST SEVERAL WEEKS.	
			12:15pm	WIFE VISITED AND PATIENT	
				BECAME QUITE EMOTIONAL.	
				DENIES PAIN BUT GRIMACES	
				OCCASIONALLY AS IF IN PAIN.	
				MONITOR SHOWS OCCASIONAL	
	SOD. LUMINAL gr. 2 I.M.	12:30		P.V.C. DR. BENTLEY	
	PULSE RATE 100	1:00	1:00 pm	SEEMS CALMER.	
	URINE SPECIMEN TO LAB.			VOIDED 300 cc CLEAR	
				AMBER URINE.	
			2:00 pm	STATES HE IS HUNGRY,	
				BROTH AND JELLO TAKEN	
				WITH GOOD APPETITE.	
				DOES NOT LIKE	
				BEING FED.	

FIG. 4–3. (*Continued*) Chart for a 24-hour period, including 8-hour summary statements.

b. Rhythm—normal sinus
　　　　sinus bradycardia
　　　　nodal
　　　　sinus tachycardia
　　　　supraventricular
　　　　ectopic atrial
　　　　block

	NURSES NOTES	COR. I. - C.C.U. BROWN, CHARLES 201000 M45 3456127 M.S. BENTLEY -H-		

DATE	MEDICATION AND TREATMENTS	HOUR	TIME	OBSERVATIONS	DOCTOR'S VISITS
10/4/69			3:00 PM	SLEEPING.	
	RHYTHM STRIP TAKEN		3:30	NORMAL SINUS RHYTHM	
		3:30 PM		RATE 100 P-R 0.2	
				VERY OCCASIONAL P.V.C.	
				DISPLAYS ANXIETY WITH	
				TENDENCY TO DENY	
				SYMPTOMS. PAIN RELIEVED	
				BY M.S. CALMED BY	
				SOD LUMINAL.	
				INTAKE : 400cc ORAL 200cc I.V	
				OUTPUT : 300cc	
				P. Kowalczyk R.N.	
	V.S. 112/90 - 100 - 22	4ᵃ	4:00 PM	WOULD LIKE TO GET UP TO	
	TEMP. 98.6			BATHROOM. NEED FOR BEDREST	
	A/R 100			EXPLAINED AS WELL AS	
				DR. BENTLEY'S PROGRAM	
				OF INCREASING ACTIVITY.	
				APPEARS TO BE MORE	
				CALM.	
			4:10	VOIDED 300cc. SEEMS TO	
				BE MORE INTERESTED	
				IN SURROUNDINGS.	
			5:00	LIQUID DIET TAKEN WELL.	
	B.P. 100/88	5ᵃ	7:00	WIFE VISITING. SHE AND	
	PHENOBARB gr. 1/4	6ᵃ		PATIENT SEEM MORE	
	B.P. 116/88			ASSURED.	
	98.2 - 114 - 22	8ᵃ	8:00	P.M. CARE. VOIDED 200 cc	
	NEMBUTAL gr. 3/4	9ᵃ	11:00	INTAKE: 600cc ORAL, 100cc IV	
				OUTPUT : 500cc	
	ECG RHYTHM STRIP	11ᵃ		NORMAL SINUS RHYTHM,	
				RATE 96	
				PR INTERVAL 0.2	
				M. Davis R.N.	

NURSES NOTES

FIG. 4–3. (*Continued*) Chart for a 24-hour period, including 8-hour summary statements.

premature beats with focus of origin idioventricular, etc.
   c. P-R interval
   d. Changes from previous strip—QRS, S-T segment, T wave, etc.
2. Summary of patient's day (any significant change from previous day)
3. Response to activity tolerance, especially as activities are increased

DATE	MEDICATION AND TREATMENTS	HOUR	TIME	OBSERVATIONS	DOCTOR'S VISITS
10/5/69			12–3:00	SLEPT WELL. GROANS IN SLEEP OCCASIONALLY. MONITOR PATTERN STABLE.	
	B.P. 116/90	3:00	3:00AM	WAKEFUL. WORRIED. ABOUT HIS CONDITION. BACK RUB, LOW CAL. GINGER ALE, REASSURANCE VOIDED 200cc CLEAR AMBER.	
			4–6:00	SLEEPING SOUNDLY. BREAKFAST HELD FOR F.B.S. ENZYMES AND ECG ORDERED	
			6:00	INTAKE: 100cc ORAL 200 I.V. OUTPUT: 200cc	
	B.P. 116/90	7:00		24 HOUR INTAKE: 1600cc OUTPUT: 1000cc	
	ECG RHYTHM STRIP RUN		7:00	NORMAL SINUS RHYTHM AT A RATE OF 90. WITH RARE P.V.C. P–R 0.2. A FAIRLY GOOD NIGHT.	
				M. Smith R.N.	

FIG. 4–3. (*Continued*) Chart for a 24-hour period,
including 8-hour summary statements.

4. Presence or absence of chest pain
5. Presence or absence of calf pain to touch or dorsiflection
6. Emotional status (degree of anxiety: reaction to diagnosis, stay in coronary care unit, visitors, or other)

An example of charting for a 24-hour period, including 8-hour summary statements, is shown in Figure 4–3.

Figure 4–4 shows an example of a nursing care plan check list.

	CHARGE PLATE
CORONARY CARE UNIT **CHECK SHEET FOR CARE**	

PERSONAL HYGIENE		OBSERVATIONS	
No bath—Nurse washes face		BP _____ time daily	
and hands	_____	Right arm	_____
Partial bath—Patient washes		Left arm	_____
face and hands	_____		
Complete bed bath	_____	TPR _____ times daily	
Tub bath or shower	_____	Temp. Oral	_____
Oral Hygiene		Rectal	_____
by others	_____	Pulse Radial	_____
by self	_____	Apical	_____
Shaving/Combing Hair			
by others	_____	POSITIONING	
by self	_____	Turn and position	
EXERCISE/ACTIVITY		by self	_____
No exercise	_____	by others	_____
Passive range of motion	_____		
Active range of motion	_____	POSITION OF BED	
Reaching for objects at		Contour	_____
bedside	_____	Semi-sitting	_____
none at all	_____	Sitting	_____
by self	_____		
Chair _____ daily		FEEDING	
for _____ length of time		Fed by others	_____
Walk _____ times daily		Assistance with feeding	_____
for _____ distance		Feeds self	_____
with assistance	_____	Avoid extremely hot or	
DIVERSIONAL ACTIVITY		cold fluids yes	_____
TV	yes _____	no	_____
	no _____	ELIMINATION	
Radio	yes _____	Urinal standing at bedside	_____
	no _____	Bedside commode	
VISITORS		BM only	_____
No visitors	_____	PRN	_____
Family visits only	_____	With assistance	_____
No restriction on visitors	_____	BRP	
Phone restrictions		With assistance	_____
Outgoing	_____		
Incoming	_____	(Signature of M.D.)	

FIGURE 4–4

A sample discharge sheet to be completed by the attending physician is shown in Figure 4–5.

CORONARY CARE UNIT
DISCHARGE SHEET

CHARGE PLATE

DATE: _____

TIME: _____

CHAIR: _____ AMBULATORY: _____ STRETCHER: _____
TRANSFER TO: _____
BLOOD PRESSURE: _____ TEMPERATURE: _____
PULSE APICAL: _____ RADIAL: _____
RESPIRATION DYSPNEA: _____ RALES: _____
EDEMA: _____
MEDICATIONS
   1. Digitalis (type) _____
      _____
   2. Antiarrhythmia _____
      _____
   3. Anticoagulant _____
      _____
   4. Diuretics _____
      _____
   5. Vasodilator _____
      _____
   6. Vasopressor _____
      _____
   7. Others _____

DIAGNOSIS: _____ INFARCTION LOCATION: _____
MAJOR ARRHYTHMIAS: _____
_____
_____

MINOR ARRHYTHMIAS: _____
_____
_____

MAJOR COMPLICATIONS: _____
_____
_____

MINOR COMPLICATIONS: _____
_____
_____

SIGNIFICANT BLOOD CHEMISTRY: _____
_____
_____
_____
_____
(Signature of M.D.)

FIGURE 4–5

REFERENCES AND BIBLIOGRAPHY

Coronary Care Unit Manual. Detroit, The Grace Hospital, 1968.

A Facility Designed for Coronary Care. Public Health Service Publication No. 930-D-19. Washington, D.C., U.S. Dept. of Health, Education and Welfare, 1965.

Lown, B., and Shillingford, J. P.: Symposium on Coronary Care Units. New York, Reuben H. Donnelley, 1967.

5 THE CORONARY CARE UNIT

The coronary care unit should be established as a separate area within the hospital. Rooms within the unit should permit maximum observation of the patients by the nurse, but should also provide privacy for the patients. Partitions between the beds prevent patients from being disturbed by activities in other rooms. Such separation is necessary since the stress induced by crisis activities with another patient may precipitate premature contractions. Figure 5–1 shows a well-designed coronary care unit.

A central panel console at the nursing station, as shown in Figure 5–2, includes an oscilloscope and a heart-rate meter with audiovisual alarm, ECG write-out and memory loop connected to each patient unit.

Although the unit is fully equipped with electronic devices to monitor the patient, its value depends upon the competence of the personnel using it.

Within the coronary care unit, the patient's room, as shown in Figure 5–3, is not only equipped with sophisticated instruments for the treatment of his physical illness, but also is attractive enough to be conducive to his psychological comfort.

EQUIPMENT IN THE PATIENT'S ROOM

1. A special bed with removable head- and foot-boards to provide easy accessibility to the patient in emergency situations
2. Wall equipment
   a. Oxygen outlet with flow meter and humidifier
   b. Suction outlet with regulator, pressure gauge and vacuum bottle
   c. Several examination lights
   d. Electrical outlets
   e. TV and radio earphone jacks

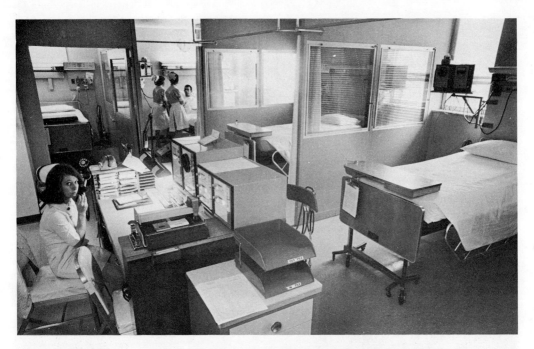

FIG. 5–1. A coronary care unit.

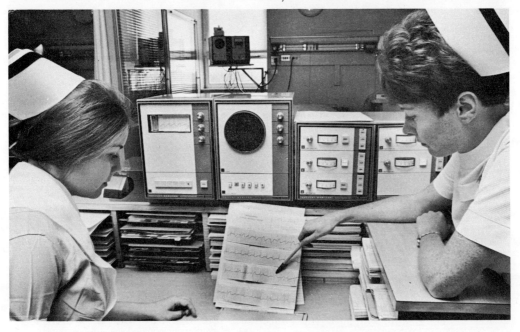

FIG. 5–2. Nursing station panel console in a coronary care unit.

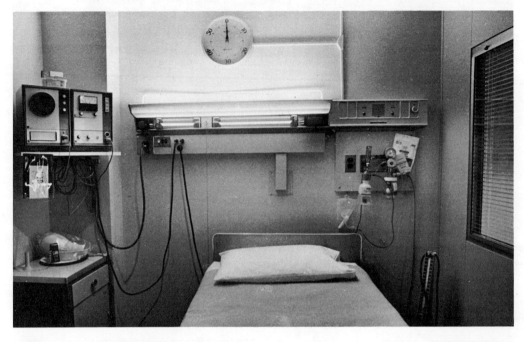

Fig. 5–3. Patient's room.

  f. Shelf to contain
   (1) transvenous catheters
   (2) disposable electrode kits
   (3) nasal catheters and masks
   (4) airway
  g. Sphygmomanometer
 3. Ceiling-mounted equipment
  a. Intravenous rods on track
  b. TV set with remote control
 4. Mounted monitor equipment
  a. Oscilloscope with an ECG memory loop
  b. Heart-rate meter with high-low-rate alarm system
  c. Pacemaker (internal-external)
 5. Clipboard at foot of bed containing
  a. Admission check-off sheet
  b. Blood-pressure graph
  c. Intake-output sheet

PATIENT MONITORING SYSTEM

To give meaning to the concept of intensive care and to prevent cardiac crisis, an electronic monitoring system is a necessary component.

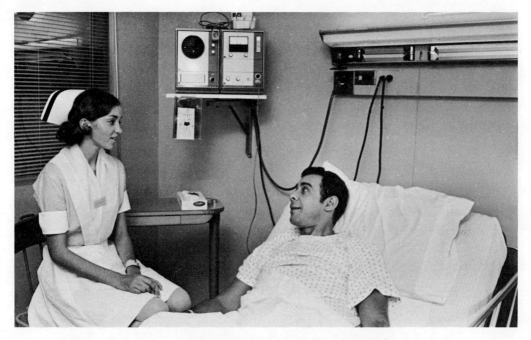

Fɪɢ. 5–4. Patient console system.

Such equipment, illustrated in Figure 5–4, augments observation of the patient's vital signs and enhances the nurse's skills in giving effective, preventive care to the patient.

The patient monitoring system is effective only when the coronary care unit is staffed with perceptive, knowledgeable nurses who are clinical specialists. The nurse is at the bedside during major clinical events and must therefore be prepared to initiate treatment for resuscitation and for the reversal of death-producing arrhythmias. Frequently, crisis intervention is required and the nurse cannot wait for the arrival of a physician.

As soon as possible after admission, the nurse attaches the ECG skin electrodes to the patient's chest and adjusts the monitor. At the same time, she assesses the cardiac status of the patient and determines whether or not he is in distress. After the monitor is attached, a rhythm strip is recorded. The nurse must be alert for any arrhythmias and must initiate the treatment program. She also identifies the patient's emotional responses and gives support as indicated.

Before electrodes are placed, the placement sites should be prepared:

1. Remove hair from each site, clearing areas 5-inches in diameter.

2. Remove surface skin oil, dead skin and moisture with acetone or alcohol, and dry thoroughly.

To reduce irritation, electrode sites should be changed every 24 hours. Recommended electrode sites are:

1. The right-arm monitoring electrode is placed below the right clavicle, midway between the shoulder and the upper sternum.
2. The left-leg monitoring electrode is placed on the interior left axillary line over the eighth and ninth ribs.
3. The right-leg ground electrode is placed on the interior right axillary line over the eighth and ninth ribs.
4. The left-arm electrode is placed below the left clavicle and is used with the lead-select switch only.

The skin electrodes pick up the electrical impulse originating in the patient's heart and direct it into an ECG amplifier. The signal is approximately one millivolt; the ECG amplifier increases this signal a thousand times, from one millivolt to one volt. After the ECG wave form has been amplified, it is displayed on the oscilloscope.

In addition to the standard monitoring leads I, II, and III, some monitors are equipped with a lead-select switch to display the unipolar limb leads and the unipolar precordial leads on the ECG amplifier.

The 5-inch oscilloscope permits visual observation of the heart signal. The heart-rate meter detects the QRS complexes and displays the patient's heart rate in beats per minute. In addition, it sounds a visual and auditory alarm when there is a lead failure or if the heart rate exceeds the previously set high- or low-rate limits.

To begin monitoring the patient, the nurse turns on the ECG amplifier, connects the patient's electrodes to the cables and adjusts the ECG wave forms on the oscilloscope.

If a wandering base line appears on the oscilloscope, the patient's electrode connections should be checked. They may need additional electrode paste, or it may be necessary to change them. If there is no patient signal or if an erratic signal appears, check the patient's electrode cable connections. Be certain the patient is not attached to or touching any ungrounded equipment.

If false QRS beats appear, check and adjust the sensitivity setting; then check the patient's signal on the oscilloscope. If the sensitivity of the monitor is set too high, portions of the cardiac cycle may register tall enough to trigger the rate counter, and thus trigger a false high-rate alarm.

False low-rate alarms may be due to detached electrodes if the monitor system is not equipped with a lead-fail alarm or, if the sensitivity of the monitor is not adjusted high enough, R waves may not display with sufficient height to trigger the rate-counting mechanism and thus trigger a low-rate alarm.

Occasionally the recommended electrode placement site will not demonstrate a satisfactory P wave. It then becomes necessary to experiment with moving the electrodes slightly in one direction or another. The Welch electrode (the suction-cup type used in the V leads of the full-scale ECG) becomes a useful tool in this hunt for a P wave because it eliminates the need to tape the electrode to the chest wall with each move. When a satisfactory P wave is found, the regular electrode can then be taped in place at that site.

False high-rate alarms may be triggered by muscle contractions which are registered on the monitor as R waves, and thus seemingly indicate a high pulse rate.

If equipment is ungrounded, it causes electrical interference and presents a severe electrical hazard to the patient, who is grounded through the monitoring electrodes.

CRASH CART EQUIPMENT

For emergency situations, the coronary care unit should have the following equipment assembled on a cart:

1. Defibrillator with R wave synchronizer to terminate life-threatening arrhythmias
2. Pacemaker, if not included in monitor, to be used for ventricular standstill
3. Automatic rotating tourniquet machine to be used in acute pulmonary edema
4. Heart–lung resuscitator for use in cardiac standstill
5. Emergency drugs with syringes and needles
6. Endotracheal tubes
7. Venous cut-down tray
8. Tracheotomy tray
9. Manual breathing bag
10. Positive-pressure breathing apparatus

ELECTRICAL DEFIBRILLATOR

The defibrillator was designed to deliver a high-voltage shock of brief duration through the chest wall to terminate ventricular fibrillation.

Kouwhenhoven designed an instrument using alternating current to terminate ventricular fibrillation. It cannot be successfully used to reverse other arrhythmias, however, because it frequently produces ventricular fibrillation. Lown designed an instrument using direct current to synchronize the short D.C. (direct current) impulse so that it avoids the vulnerable phase of the heart cycle. (This vulnerable phase precedes the peak T wave on the ECG.) The shock is administered during the down slope of the R wave in the QRS complex. Figure 5–6 shows a D.C. defibrillator.

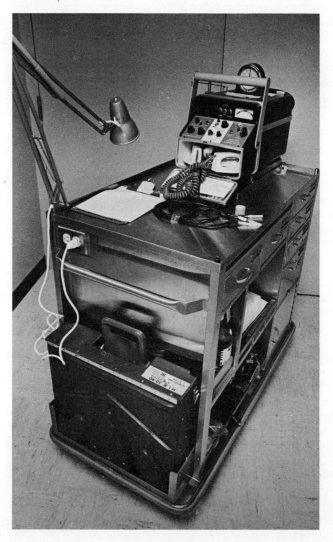

FIG. 5-5. Crash cart.

In defibrillation for ventricular fibrillation, the synchronizer must be turned off or, since there is no R wave to synchronize with, the defibrillator will not discharge. If ventricular fibrillation is associated with cardiac arrest, electrical defibrillation is the only treatment. Cardiopulmonary resuscitation measures should be maintained until immediately before defibrillation, and resumed immediately afterward if the pulse

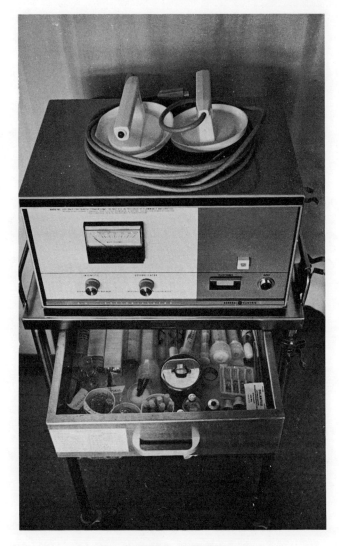

FIG. 5–6. D.C. defibrillator.

and blood pressure are not satisfactory, even if a successful response to defibrillation has been obtained.

As soon as ventricular fibrillation has been timed and confirmed on the oscilloscope, sound the physician alarm and start the automatic timer set at 2 minutes.

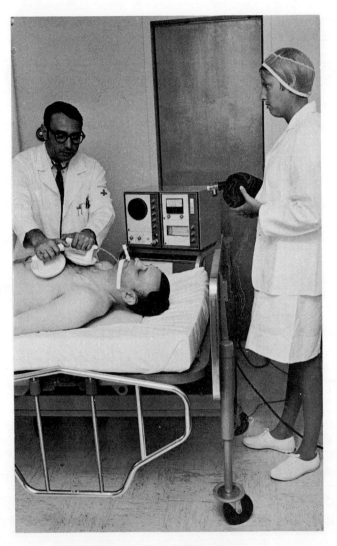

FIG. 5–7. Use of defibrillator
in cardiac resuscitation.

NURSING RESPONSIBILITIES

1. Prepare the defibrillator paddles with sufficient electrode paste. Too little paste may result in a severe burn to the patient.
2. Be sure that the skin on the patient's chest is dry. Give 100 watt-seconds with a D.C. defibrillator within 30 seconds of arrest. If suc-

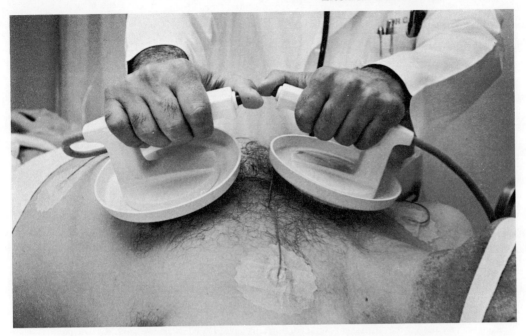

Fig. 5–8. Defibrillator paddle placement.

cessive tries are needed, increase the voltage to 200, 300 and 400 watt-seconds with successive attempts.

3. *Defibrillate the patient if the physician has not arrived within 2 minutes.* Defibrillation within 30 seconds is much more likely to be successful because of better myocardial oxygenation. When hospital policy requires the nurse to wait 2 minutes for the physician before she can proceed with defibrillation, it is imperative that cardiac massage and assisted respiration be continued from the moment of arrest to the moment of defibrillation.

4. Hold the paddles tightly against the chest wall with about 30 pounds of pressure. One paddle is placed at the apex of the heart; the other is placed at the second intercostal space, as shown in Figures 5–7 and 5–8.

5. Avoid touching the patient, bed or other contact surfaces when the trigger is fired, and use a code such as "Hit it" or "All hands off" to alert other personnel.

6. Fire the trigger as soon as possible.

7. Check monitor to see if fibrillation has terminated. If not, repeat shock.

8. Check monitor and observe state of consciousness; if defibrillation is successful, the patient awakens within one minute and the pulse is palpable.

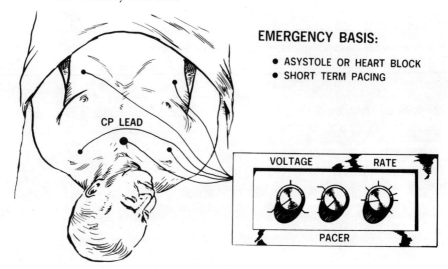

FIG. 5–9. Pacer module.

Medications available for use include:

1. Sodium bicarbonate to correct acidosis, which inhibits cardiac resuscitation by depressing myocardial function and reducing cardiac output
2. Epinephrine to increase the force of myocardial contraction
3. Vasopressors such as Levophed or Aramine to maintain blood pressure
4. Antiarrhythmia drugs such as Pronestyl to reduce myocardial irritability

Pulmonary ventilation must be maintained. Endotracheal intubation should be performed as soon as possible, and oxygen started.

The patient's response to therapy should be carefully noted and recorded.

When fibrillation is converted to standstill, slow idioventricular rhythm or extreme bradycardia, the external pacemaker is used to stimulate the heart by a series of electric shocks.

EXTERNAL PACING

The external pacemaker is designed to provide short-term pacing on an emergency basis in cardiac arrest or heart block. Most patient monitoring systems include a pacer module, shown in Figure 5–9, designed to function automatically as soon as the low-rate alarm sounds. These may also be operated manually.

The pacemaker electrode (C/P) may be attached to the patient's chest wall when the monitoring electrodes are positioned at the time of admission to the coronary care unit. When the external pacer module is automatically set, it may be activated by a false alarm of the monitor. This is a frightening experience for the patient. The pacer electrode is normally placed on the sternum or over the apex of the heart.

The pace pulse is applied to the patient's heart through the external pacer electrode (C/P) and the right-leg electrode, which is the ground electrode. The voltage control is used to vary the voltage of the pace pulse from 50 to 150 volts. The rate regulator is used to set the number of pace pulses delivered to the patient. These may range from 45 to 150 pulses per minute.

Use of the external pacemaker is indicated in ventricular asystole or heart block. It is a quick, effective method of re-initiating cardiac action. External pacing is painful and anxiety producing, and is continued for only brief periods until endocardial pacing is accomplished under fluoroscopic control. Because of the distress which external pacing causes the patient, the current trend in emergency pacing situations is to manipulate a slender unipolar electrode catheter into the ventricle through a large bore needle placed in the chest wall. The catheter is then attached to an external pulse generator.

NURSING RESPONSIBILITIES
1. Alert physician.
2. Determine basic cardiac rhythm on the ECG before electrical pacing.
3. Set pulse rate.

When the low-rate alarm sounds, make a rapid assessment of the patient's clinical condition. With ventricular asystole the patient immediately loses consciousness since circulation has stopped. Alert the physician and set the timer.

Check for ventricular asystole or ventricular fibrillation on the oscilloscope because the resuscitative measures will differ.

In Adams-Stokes heart block there are no ventricular contractions and, consequently, there is no heartbeat.

The ground electrode is located on the patient's right interior axillary line over the eighth and ninth ribs.

If the pacemaker has been set on the automatic position, it will start pacing when the low-rate alarm sounds. If it is not set on automatic, start the pacemaker manually. Do not wait for the physician.

Turn the rate knob to 70 and then turn on the voltage as indicated until effective heart contractions are detected by palpation.

If the heartbeat has not been restored within one minute, begin cardiopulmonary resuscitative measures.

DRUGS AND SOLUTIONS USUALLY STOCKED IN THE CORONARY CARE UNIT

The drug and solution inventories (Tables 5–1 and 5–2) which follow were established for a 5-bed coronary care unit. The content and quantity

TABLE 5–1. DRUG INVENTORY

CATEGORY	GENERIC NAME	PROPRIETARY NAME	DOSAGE FORM	UNIT SIZE	STRENGTH	QUANTITY
Analgesics	Propoxyphene HCl	Darvon	cap.		32 mg.	10
	Propoxyphene HCl	Darvon	cap.		65 mg.	10
	Pentazocine lactate	Talwin	amp.	1 cc.	30 mg./cc.	10
	Acetaminophen	Tylenol	tab.		325 mg.	10
Antiarrhythmics	Lidocaine	Xylocaine	vial	5 cc.	2%	10
	Lidocaine	Xylocaine	vial	50 cc.	20 mg./cc.	10
	Procainamide HCl	Pronestyl	vial	10 cc.	100 mg./cc.	20
	Procainamide HCl	Pronestyl	cap.		250 mg.	20
	Quinidine sulfate		tab.		3 gr.	20
	Quinidine gluconate		vial	10 cc.	0.08 Gm./cc.	2
	Sodium diphenylhydantoin	Dilantin	vial		250 mg.	6
	Sodium diphenylhydantoin	Dilantin	cap.		100 mg.	6
Antibiotic	Buffered potassium penecillin G for I.V.		vial		20,000,000 U	3
	Buffered potassium penicillin G for I.V. or I.M.		vial		1,000,000 U	3
	Sodium ampicillin for I.V. or I.M.	Penbritin-S	vial		1,000 mg.	3
	Sodium Cephalothin for I.V. or I.M.	Keflin	vial		1,000 mg.	3
Anticoagulant	Bishydroxycoumarin	Dicumarol	tab.		25 mg.	3
	Bishydroxycoumarin	Dicumarol	tab.		50 mg.	3
	Sodium warfarin	Coumadin	tab.		2 mg.	6
	Sodium warfarin	Coumadin	tab.		2.5 mg.	6
	Sodium warfarin	Coumadin	tab.		5 mg.	6
	Sodium warfarin	Coumadin	tab.		25 mg.	3
	Sodium heparin inj.	Lipo-Hepin	vial	1 cc.	10,000 U/cc.	10

Category	Generic name	Brand name	Form	Volume	Strength	Quantity
Anticoagulant antagonists	Protamine sulfate		amp.			2
	Phytonadione U.S.P.	Mephyton	amp.	1 cc.	1% 10 mg./cc.	2
Anticonvulsant	Sodium amobarbital	Amytal sodium	amp.		250 mg.	2
	Sodium diphenylhydantoin	Dilantin	vial		250 mg.	6
	Diazepam	Valium injectable	amp.	2 cc.	5 mg./cc.	6
Antidiabetic	Insulin	Regular Iletin	vial	10 cc.	80 U/cc.	1
Antihistamine	Diphenhydramine HCl	Benadryl	amp.	1 cc.	50 mg./cc.	4
Antinauseant & tranquilizer	Chlorpromazine HCl	Thorazine	amp.	2 cc.	25 mg./cc.	3
	Dimenhydrinate	Dramamine	vial	5 cc.	50 mg./cc.	1
	Hydroxyzine HCl	Vistaril	amp.	2 cc.	50 mg./cc.	3
	Prochlorperazine	Compazine	amp.	2 cc.	5 mg./cc.	3
	Promazine HCl	Sparine	vial	2 cc.	50 mg./cc.	3
	Promethazine HCl	Phenergan	amp.	1 cc.	25 mg./cc.	3
	Trimethobenzamide HCl	Tigan	amp.	2 cc.	100 mg./cc.	2
Blocking agents	Atropine sulfate		amp.	0.5 cc.	1/150 gr.	20
	Phenoxybenzamine HCl	Dibenzyline	cap.		10 mg.	2
	Phentolamine	Regitine	amp.		5 mg.	5
	Propanolol HCl	Inderal	amp.	1 cc.	1 mg./cc.	6
	Propanolol HCl	Inderal	tab.		10 mg.	10
	Propanolol HCl	Inderal	tab.		40 mg.	6
	Succinylcholine HCl	Quelicin	vial	10 cc.	20 mg./cc.	2
Bronchodilator	Aminophylline U.S.P.		amp.	10 cc.	250 mg./10 cc.	4
	Aminophylline U.S.P.		amp.	20 cc.	500 mg./20 cc.	4
Buffering agents	Ringer's lactate Tromethamine with electrolytes	THAM-E	amp. vial	20 cc.	0.3 Molar when dilute in 1000 cc. sterile water	1
Coronary vasodilators	Glyceryl trinitrate (nitroglycerin)		tab.		1/200 gr.	100
	Glyceryl trinitrate (nitroglycerin)		tab.		1/150 gr.	100
	Glyceryl trinitrate (nitroglycerin)		tab.		1/100 gr.	100

TABLE 5–1. DRUG INVENTORY (continued)

Category	Generic Name	Proprietary Name	Dosage Form	Unit Size	Strength	Quantity
Diagnostic	Phentolamine	Regitine	amp.		5 mg.	5
	Sodium dehydrocholate	Decholin Sodium	amp.	5 cc.	200 mg./5 cc.	1
Digitalis	Deslanoside inj.	Cedilanid	amp.	2 cc.	0.2 mg./cc.	10
	Digitoxin	Crystodigin	tab.		0.2 mg.	6
	Digitoxin	Crystodigin	amp.	1 cc.	0.2 mg./cc.	5
	Digoxin	Lanoxin	amp.	2 cc.	0.25 mg./cc.	5
	Digoxin	Lanoxin	tab.		0.25 mg.	5
Diuretics	Acetazolamide	Diamox	vial		500 mg.	1
	Furosemide	Lasix	amp.	2 cc.	10 mg./cc.	2
	Mannitol N.F.		amp.	50 cc.	12.5 Gm./cc.	2
	Meralluride inj. U.S.P.	Mercuhydrin	amp.	2 cc.		4
	Sodium ethacrynate	Sodium Lyovac Edecrin	vial		50 mg.	5
Electrolytes	Calcium chloride		amp.	10 cc.	1 Gm.	10
	Calcium gluconate		amp.	10 cc.	1 Gm.	5
	Potassium chloride		amp.	20 cc.	40 mEq.	5
	Potassium chloride		amp.	20 cc.	20 mEq.	5
	Sodium bicarbonate		amp.	50 cc.	3.75 Gm.	20
Hypoglycemia	Dextrose 50%		amp.	50 cc.	25 Gm.	3
	Glucagon for inj.		vial	1 cc.	1 mg.	6
Hypotensives	Phenoxybenzamine HCl	Dibenzyline	cap.		10 mg.	1
	Reserpine	Serpasil	amp.	2 cc.	2.5 mg./cc.	1
	Trimethaphan	Arfonad	amp.	10 cc.	50 mg./cc.	1
Local anesthetic	Lidocaine HCl	Xylocaine HCl	amp.	2 cc.	2%	4
Narcotics	Codeine phosphate		amp.	1 cc.	½ gr.	20
	Morphine sulfate		amp.	1 cc.	¼ gr.	20
	Morphine sulfate		amp.	1 cc.	⅙ gr.	20
	Meperidine HCl	Demerol	amp.	1 cc.	100 mg./cc.	20

Category	Generic name	Trade name	Form			Quantity
Narcotic antagonist	Nalorphine HCl	Nalline	amp.	2 cc.	10 mg.	3
Ophthalmological	Methylcellulose in isotonic solution	Tearisol	lacravial	0.5 fl. oz.		1
Psycho stimulant	Methylergonovine maleate	Methergine	amp.	1 cc.	0.2 mg./cc.	2
Respiratory stimulant	Ethamivan	Emivan	amp.	2 cc.	50 mg./cc.	2
Sedatives	Chloral betaine	Beta-Chlor	tab.		7½ gr.	6
	Glutethimide	Doriden	tab.		0.5 Gm.	6
	Sodium pentobarbital	Nembutal sodium	cap.		100 mg.	20
	Sodium pentobarbital inj.	Nembutal sodium inj.	amp.	2 cc.	1½ gr./2 cc.	2
	Sodium secobarbital	Seconal sodium	cap.		1½ gr.	20
	Sodium secobarbital inj.	Seconal sodium inj.	amp.		250 mg.	2
Steroids	Hydrocortisone sodium succinate	Solu-Cortef	vial	2 cc.	100 mg./2 cc.	4
	Methylprednisolone sodium succinate	Solu-Medrol	vial	1 cc.	40 mg.	2
	Methylprednisolone sodium succinate	Solu-Medrol	vial	2 cc.	125 mg.	2
Vasopressors	Angiotensin amide	Hypertensin	vial		2.5 mg.	1
	Epinephrine	Adrenalin	amp.	1 cc.	1:1000	6
	Isoproterenol HCl	Isuprel HCl	amp.	1 cc.	0.2 mg./cc.	10
	Isoproterenol HCl	Isuprel HCl	amp.	5 cc.	1 mg./5 cc.	10
	Levarterenol bitartrate	Levophed bitartrate	amp.	4 cc.	0.2%	20
	Metaraminol bitartrate	Aramine bitartrate	amp.	1 cc.	10 mg./cc.	6
	Metaraminol bitartrate	Aramine bitartrate	amp.	10 cc.	10 mg./cc.	6
	Methoxamine HCl	Vasoxyl	amp.	1 cc.	20 mg.	1
	Phenylephrine HCl	Neo-Synephrine HCl	amp.	1 cc.	10 mg.	1

of stock should be altered in accordance with the speed with which required medications can be obtained from a central pharmacy.

Good practice dictates that, whenever possible, fresh unit dosages be used in preference to multiple-dose containers. All items stocked should be handled in compliance with state and federal drug-control regulations.

The drugs in Tables 5–1 and 5–2 have been categorized according to their major therapeutic effect. If a drug has more than one major therapeutic effect, it may be listed more than once.

The charge nurse should be given the responsibility of a daily check of the drug inventory. This can be done quickly if drugs are stored alphabetically in a medication-drawer cabinet.

TABLE 5–2. INTRAVENOUS SOLUTION INVENTORY

DRUG	STRENGTH	VEHICLE	UNIT SIZE	QUANTITY
Dextran 75	6% W/V	Normal saline	1000 cc.	1
Dextran 75	6% W/V	Normal saline	500 cc.	1
Dextran 75	6% W/V	Distilled water-5% dextrose	500 cc.	1
LM Dextran 40	10% W/V	Normal saline	500 cc.	1
LM Dextran 40	10% W/V	5% dextrose-distilled water	500 cc.	1
Glucose	5%	Distilled water	1000 cc.	2
Glucose	5%	Distilled water	500 cc.	4
Glucose	5%	Distilled water	250 cc.	4
Glucose	5%	Normal saline	1000 cc.	2
Glucose	5%	Normal saline	500 cc.	1
Glucose	5%	⅓ normal saline	1000 cc.	2
Glucose	5%	⅓ normal saline	500 cc.	2
Glucose	5%	½ normal saline	500 cc.	2
Glucose	5%	Lactated Ringer's solution	1000 cc.	2
Glucose-Alcohol	5% each	Distilled water	1000 cc.	1
Glucose	10%	Distilled water	1000 cc.	2
Glucose	10%	Normal saline	1000 cc.	1
Osmitrol	5%	Distilled water	1000 cc.	1
Osmitrol	10%	Distilled water	1000 cc.	1
Osmitrol	20%	Distilled water	1000 cc.	1
		Normal saline	1000 cc.	1
		Normal saline	500 cc.	1
		Normal saline	250 cc.	1

REFERENCES AND BIBLIOGRAPHY

Adkins, P. C., and Byers, W. S.: Indication for cardiac pacemaking. A.O.R.N., *8:*48-56, (Sept.) 1968.

Beland, I.: Clinical Nursing. pp. 561-731. New York, Macmillan, 1965.

Bernreiter, M.: Electrocardiography. ed. 2. Philadelphia, J. B. Lippincott, 1963.

Brunner, L. S., Emerson, C. P., Ferguson, L. K., and Suddarth, D. S.: Textbook of Medical-Surgical Nursing. ed. 2. pp. 359-392. Philadelphia, J. B. Lippincott, 1970.

Friedberg, C. K.: Diseases of the Heart. ed. 3. pp. 219-242, 284-304, 443-474, 483-575, 583-628, 643-693, 706-763, 770-791, 866-922. Philadelphia, W. B. Saunders, 1966.

Hanchett, E. S., and Johnson, R. A.: Early signs of congestive heart failure. Am. J. Nurs., *68:*1456-1461, (July) 1968.

Humphries, J.: Treatment of heart block with artificial pacemakers. Mod. Conc. Cardiov. Dis., *33:*857-861, (June) 1964.

Hurst, J. W., and Logue, R. R.: The Heart. pp. 224-234, 239-282, 285-341, 350-362. New York, McGraw-Hill, 1966.

Lown, B.: Intensive heart care. Sci. Am., *219:*19-27, (July) 1968.

MacBryde, C.: Signs and Symptoms. ed. 4. pp. 262-308, 335. Philadelphia, J. B. Lippincott, 1964.

Meltzer, L. E., *et al.:* Intensive Coronary Care—A Manual for Nurses. CCU Fund, Philadelphia Presbyterian Hospital, 1965.

Rodman, M., and Smith, D.: Pharmacology and Drug Therapy in Nursing. pp. 275-368. Philadelphia, J. B. Lippincott, 1968.

Shafer, K. N., Sawyer, J. R., McClusky, A. M., and Beck, E. L.: Medical-Surgical Nursing. ed. 4. pp. 317-346, 358-361. St. Louis, C. V. Mosby, 1967.

Smith, D. W., and Gips, C. D.: Care of the Adult Patient. ed. 2. pp. 529-580, 627-637. Philadelphia, J. B. Lippincott, 1966.

Sowton, E.: Cardiac pacemakers and pacing. Mod. Conc. Cardiov. Dis., *36:*31-36, (June) 1967.

Unger, P. N.: Electrical conversion of cardiac arrhythmias. Am. J. Nurs., *66:*1962-1965, (Sept.) 1966.

Wood, P.: Diseases of the Heart and Circulation. ed. 3. Philadelphia, J. B. Lippincott, 1968.

6 PSYCHOLOGICAL RESPONSES IN THE CORONARY CARE UNIT

The admission of the patient to the coronary care unit is a dramatic event. Its impact is not lost on the patient. Beginning with the attack of crushing, intense pain, his life is suddenly altered, indeed threatened. Vaguely he remembers the doctor, the shot in the arm, the ambulance.

The admission procedure is routine for the nurse but strange and frightening to the patient. For the patient in acute distress, the nurse must identify priority needs and act promptly to meet them:

1. Notify the medical resident.
2. Apply monitor, assess the heart rhythm and record an ECG tracing.
3. Start nasal oxygen if indicated.
4. Record temperature, blood pressure and apical-radial pulse.
5. Start the treatment program for any complication.

Not only must the nurse make a rapid assessment of the patient's physical condition, but she must also assess his emotional state.

1. What is he thinking about?
2. How anxious is he?
3. What does his facial expression reveal?
4. Does he lie rigidly in bed?
5. Is he mentally alert or confused?
6. Are his eyes restless? Do they dart about, unable to stay focused on anything for more than a second?
7. Does he watch every move the nurse makes?
8. Does he talk rapidly or slowly? Is the pitch of his voice high?
9. Does he think he's going to die?

Emotional factors enter into every patient's illness; typically he feels some anxiety about his condition. The patient with a myocardial infarc-

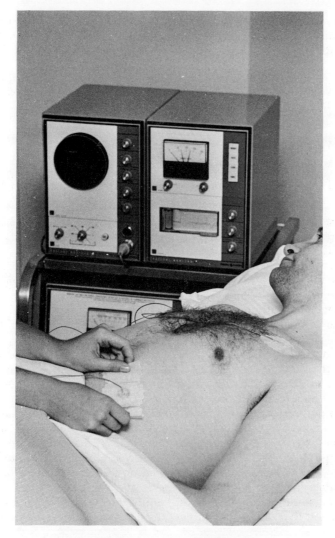

FIG. 6–1. A nurse placing electrodes.

tion feels that his life is threatened and is deeply concerned about his condition, fearful that he may die at any moment. The way the nurse responds to these feelings will greatly influence his recovery.

A positive reassuring attitude is essential when caring for a patient with a myocardial infarction. However, this does not imply giving the patient a false reassurance by saying, "Don't worry, everything will be fine." During the initial interaction between the nurse and the patient, a therapeutic climate is built upon trust and understanding. Dialogue between the nurse and patient may progress along this line:

PATIENT: Where am I? What happened to me?

NURSE: You are in a special unit where we can watch you closely. Do you still have pain? Any trouble breathing?

PATIENT: Where is my wife?

NURSE: Your wife may see you in a few moments.

PATIENT: What are you doing to my chest?

NURSE: I'm attaching wires to your chest so that we can watch your heartbeat on a screen.

How should the nurse answer the patient's question, "Am I going to die?" She simply states, "I don't know, but we have a specially trained staff and the equipment to watch you closely."

The nurse should assess the patient's degree of anxiety. It is extremely rare that apprehension and anxiety are not present after a myocardial infarction. Each individual reacts differently. Some patients are frank in their comments, while others feel so threatened that they choose denial as a defense mechanism. Most patients fall somewhere between the two extremes.

The nurse should display an alert, gentle and compassionate attitude. Answer the patient's questions briefly. If he asks none, answer his unspoken questions. Do not overwhelm him with information which he will not be able to assimilate.

An important factor in the patient's recovery is his family and their response to his illness. They also need the same information and consideration given to the patient. Calm explanations reduce fear of the unit and its equipment. The family should be given a coronary care unit information pamphlet which indicates the visiting schedule, location of waiting rooms, cafeteria service, phone calls and so on.

The nurse should explain to the family the concept of intensive coronary care and that the patient will get the best nursing care possible.

REACTION TO THE ENVIRONMENT

The patient with a myocardial infarction may exhibit any number of emotional responses and the nurse must be able to identify them. All her skills based on psychiatric concepts are needed to help the patient accept his illness and plan for his recovery.

The degree of anxiety experienced by the patient is beyond the normal level if it interferes with his ability to think rationally. It dissipates his energy and, if prolonged, can overwhelm him. To reduce the patient's anxiety level:

1. Greet the patient by name, sit down at his bedside, and be available.
2. Briefly explain his illness and treatment.
3. Explain the monitor and electrodes, the alarm system and the false alarms that may occur.
4. While talking, provide openings for the patient to communicate his fears.
5. Accept his feelings by indicating that you understand why he is concerned.

Denial, anger and hostility are not unusual responses. The patient may use these responses to help control his anxiety. The nursing goal is to assist the patient to accept and to understand his illness.

1. The nurse may initiate a conversation by saying, "I can understand why you are upset by this illness."
2. Gradually encourage him to express his feelings.
3. If he chooses not to talk, it may be helpful to sit with him for 5 or 10 minutes. There are some situations where nonverbal communication is more meaningful. The nurse must learn to be comfortable in such situations and to be alert to what she is communicating as well as perceiving. If the patient feels that the nurse is interested in him, he may feel encouraged to talk.

The nurse who permits the patient to become overdependent, however, is doing him a great disservice and may be meeting her own needs at his expense. Nevertheless, it is important that the nurse offer strong support to the patient throughout the course of his illness. He needs to know that his heart is the finest pump ever created, that it is strong and has a built-in capacity for self-repair when injured.

The nurse explains the activity program planned for the patient by his physician and permits him to set his own pace of basic care.

Frequently, the patient is confused about the time and day of the week, and expresses his concern about this. The isolation of the unit and his sedation contribute to his confusion. To strengthen his comprehension of the situation:

1. A nighttime sleeping schedule should be maintained whenever possible.
2. Clocks which indicate the date and day of the week are available and should be placed in every patient unit.
3. If the patient's condition permits, use of radio or TV is helpful. The nurse should be alert to the effects such diversions may have on his heart rate and rhythm.

Depression may result from boredom and from concern about the future. Enforced dependency is difficult for most adults to accept. The nurse should explain to the patient why his activities are restricted. She should encourage the patient to establish realistic immediate and long-range goals and should discuss these with him. This facilitates attaining a major nursing goal of instilling self-confidence in the patient.

In a very short time the patient becomes aware of other patients in the unit and soon learns when they are having difficulties. He should be protected from traumatic perceptual experiences so that outside crisis activity will not produce a stress reaction in him which could precipitate an arrhythmia.

REACTION TO DISCHARGE FROM THE CORONARY CARE UNIT

The patient's stay in the coronary care unit is usually limited to 3 to 5 days. It is not unusual for patients to become dependent on the monitors and the constant nursing observation, and many are afraid to leave the unit.

The patient's reaction to his transfer from the coronary care unit will depend upon his feelings of security and the degree of understanding he has about his illness. One patient may view the transfer positively, a sign that his condition has improved. Another may view the move with feelings of anxiety and fear that may make him restless and unable to sleep.

Preparation of the patient for transfer should be included in the nursing care plan. Shortly after admission, the patient and his family should be informed how long he will be in the coronary care unit.

In some hospitals, the coronary care unit is located within another patient care unit. Ideally, patients are transferred from the coronary care unit to this unit, which is equipped with a central console monitor. In this unit, the patient wears a pocketsized transmitter and the ECG signal is relayed to the central console by telemetry. The patient is not restricted to his bed or room and may begin ambulatory activities.

The nurse from the transfer unit should be invited to the coronary care unit to meet the patient and discuss his care. This will reassure the patient that he will be cared for, and conveys the nurses' interest in his welfare. The transfer unit nurse has the opportunity to reduce the patient's anxiety level and answer any questions he may have about his new surroundings. The unspoken fears of abandonment which the patient may have can be relieved by meeting the nurse who will be concerned with the next phase of his rehabilitation.

In giving care to the patient, the nurse utilizes her knowledge, emotions, experiences, humor and insight to assess the patient and his needs.

She must realize that each patient is a unique individual who will evoke an emotional response in her. All these factors influence the patient's recovery. To get him actively involved in his recovery, the nurse should:

1. Offer broad openings for the patient to talk about his concern for the future.
2. Accept his fears as being real and legitimate feelings.
3. Help him to understand that he can still lead a productive life.
4. Assist the patient in establishing goals within the scope of his limitations.

NURSE-PATIENT RELATIONSHIPS

By his very nature, man is a social being—one who not only expresses himself but indeed arrives at fullness as a person through communication with others. It may be said that intelligent communication—communication at a meaningful level—is a mark of what it is to be a man. As a human response to persons in distress, nursing demands effective communication.

Communication often fails because a satisfactory relationship is not established. Warm responsiveness by the nurse creates a climate enabling rapport. She must be sensitive to the needs of the patient, recognizing that all behavior is meaningful. She will become emotionally involved with him to some extent—an involvement which must permit therapeutic intervention for the patient's welfare. The patient's predominant psychological needs are:

1. The need for security or protection from threat
2. The need for acceptance—for a sense of belonging
3. The need for self-expression as an outlet for his tensions and fears
4. The need to be understood
5. The need for feelings of worth; the illness may have damaged his self-esteem.

The nurse is an actor in a highly technical stage setting. Her audience, the patients, watch every expression and move. To avoid arousing anxiety in the patient, she must learn to control her emotional responses and to direct them into therapeutic channels. She must appear alert and stable to provide a beneficial, effective climate for the patient.

While setting the climate for interaction with the patient, the nurse assesses his emotional state. What emotional responses are predominant? Gradually, she helps him to start thinking in terms of how he feels. Her responses help to develop a relationship which displays her understanding of his feelings as well as her willingness to help him cope with them.

While the patient may be able to express some of his feelings, there may be others that he cannot express. The nurse should understand what it means to be suddenly admitted to a hospital. Simple, brief explanations will assist the patient to accept his environment and the dependence his illness has thrust upon him.

Rest is one of the key factors in recovery. The nurse communicates this to the patient and controls the amount of noise and other extraneous factors which may interfere with the patient's rest. Explanations reduce anxiety and make it possible for the patient to relax and rest.

PATIENT PARTICIPATION

In addition to his other needs, the patient has the need to understand his illness. He needs to know what he can do to facilitate his recovery.

Hospitalization is, in some respects, a growth and development process. Initially, the patient, like the infant, is forced to rely upon others for the satisfaction of his physical and emotional requirements. As his condition improves, he assumes more control over his environment.

Patient participation should be encouraged as soon as his condition permits. The patient may exhibit negative feelings about his recovery or be reluctant to talk about his way of life and the way he related to others. Gradually he can be encouraged to express and examine his habits and feelings so that he may understand them and, in some instances, learn to modify them.

Because of the amount of information available to the general public, most patients have some idea of what heart disease is. Hence, most of them will ask questions. The answers given require mature judgment on the part of the nurse. They must ultimately be related to the personality structure of the patient, his perspective of reality and his anxiety level.

The patient with a myocardial infarction will be on bed rest for the first 2 weeks since rest is a primary requisite in the treatment program. Thus, helping the patient accept short-range goals is essential to his recovery. He will need an explanation of bed rest and why it is required.

As the physician's program of planned activities is implemented and new activities are introduced, careful observation of the patient is important regarding chest pain, changes in pulse rate and rhythm, increase in respirations, fatigue and changes in blood pressure. His total response to activity is a significant factor in planning his program of care.

The nurse's teaching role is an important aspect of the nursing process. The teaching plan should be tailored to meet the needs of the patient; it should be implemented in terms that he understands and in a way that he will accept. The plan should include:

1. Information that he and his family need to understand the illness
2. Realistic short- and long-range goals
3. Stress on prevention of further attacks

4. Helping the patient and his family accept the leading role in his recovery

REHABILITATION

Complete recovery from a myocardial infarction to a nearly normal way of life is common. The patient soon learns that he can lead a productive life if he sets his own pace in increasing his activities with a common sense approach.

The nursing discharge plan usually includes the following instructions:

1. **Modify work load.** The amount of work that the patient is able to assume depends upon his occupation and the amount of scar tissue on the myocardium. Long, sustained work should be avoided. An extra half hour for lunch to relax in a quiet, pleasant atmosphere is beneficial. A housewife should resume her work load gradually, and learn to do things in an easy way. The American Heart Association has many pamphlets which indicate how household tasks can be simplified.

2. **Restrict activities.** Patients who experience little or no distress as they start ambulating should be encouraged to take short walks. Walking is one of the best forms of physical activity.

   Strenuous activities are to be permanently avoided since they place a strain on the heart. These include pushing a stalled car, shoveling snow, changing a tire, and similar activities.

3. **No smoking.** Smoking constricts blood vessels, increases the heart rate and raises the blood pressure. Recent government studies indicate that the morbidity rate in coronary disease is higher with smokers than nonsmokers. Continued smoking by persons with coronary disease increases the risk of another attack.

4. **Modify living pattern.** The patient should be encouraged not to take assignments from work to be completed at home. His time at home should be used for rest and participation in relaxing activities. Visits with friends should be short to avoid fatigue or excessive stimulation.

   Sexual intercourse is usually restricted for several months after recovery from infarction due to the stress it places upon circulation. In some instances, it may be restricted for a longer period.

5. **Moderate exercise.** Strenuous sports such as baseball, football, hunting and tennis should be avoided by postinfarction patients. Golf and swimming are permissible if the patient is not subject to anginal pain.

6. **Relaxing hobby.** Every individual should have at least one hobby which supplies an outlet for tension.

7. **Watch weight and diet.** All patients who have had a coronary attack should be encouraged to maintain normal weight. Heavy eating should be avoided since it may precipitate an anginal attack. A low fat diet is recommended to lower the serum cholesterol level.

REFERENCES AND BIBLIOGRAPHY

Aspects of Anxiety. Philadelphia, J. B. Lippincott, 1965.

Gordon, J. E.: Personality and Behavior. New York, Macmillan, 1963.

Klein, R. F., Kliner, V. A., Zipes, D. P., Tryoer, W. G., and Wallace, A. G.: Transfer from a coronary care unit. Arch. Intern. Med. *122*:104-108, (August) 1968.

Marmor, J.: Modern Psychoanalysis. New York, Basic Books, 1968.

Norbeck, E., et al.: The Study of Personality. New York, Holt, Rinehart and Winston, 1968.

Skipper, J. K., and Leonard, R. C.: Social Interaction and Patient Care. Philadelphia, J. B. Lippincott, 1965.

7 COMPLICATIONS OF MYOCARDIAL INFARCTION

Planned, direct observation of the patient's clinical status is essential to detect the complications which may occur with myocardial infarctions. This chapter will consider the major complications (other than the arrhythmias) for which the nursing personnel must be alert.

LEFT HEART FAILURE

Left heart failure following myocardial infarction is due to failure of the left heart to empty properly. The cardiac chambers dilate and the veins are distended and engorged by the rapidly increasing pressure.

Reduced cardiac output by the left heart, with more blood being delivered into the pulmonary circulation by the right ventricle than is removed by the left, produces pulmonary congestion and results in a rapid escape of capillary fluid into the alveoli, reducing the oxygen supply. Figure 7–1 illustrates this congestion.

Symptoms

1. Dyspnea
2. Anxiety
3. Shock

Acute pulmonary edema is characterized by a severe attack of paroxysmal dyspnea. If it occurs at night, the patient awakens suddenly, unable to breathe. He usually displays anxiety because of the oppressive sensation in his chest. The pulse is rapid and thready, and the blood pressure drops suddenly because the heart cannot fill up the arterial system as quickly as it drains.

With rapidly increasing engorgement, the interstitial and alveolar edema inhibits oxygen and carbon dioxide diffusion in the lungs, resulting

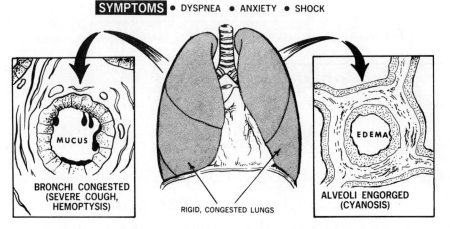

SYMPTOMS • DYSPNEA • ANXIETY • SHOCK

FIG. 7–1. Acute pulmonary edema.

in dyspnea and cyanosis. Hypoxia and carbon dioxide retention increase as pulmonary function decreases. The increased carbon dioxide will cause respiratory acidosis.

The dilated blood vessels and the collection of the mucus in the lungs make the patient cough incessantly, and often the patient's sputum is blood tinged. Respirations are moist, and audible rales are heard.

Treatment

The treatment of acute pulmonary edema consists of the following:

1. Reduction of central and total blood volume
2. Improved arterial oxygen saturation
3. Improved cardiac performance

Nursing Responsibilities

1. The nurse should be alert for symptoms of congestive failure.
2. She should be alert for dyspnea and note its progressive severity.
3. One of the first emergency measures is the application of rotating tourniquets to restrict venous return.
4. If the use of rotating tourniquets is not effective, phlebotomy may be performed to decrease the blood volume if the patient is not in shock.
5. Oxygen by mask or catheter should be started to prevent further engorgement. A positive-pressure respirator may be used to increase oxygen concentration.
6. Respiratory depressants decrease the exaggerated inspiratory effort. This exaggerated effort reduces intrathoracic pressure, thus permitting

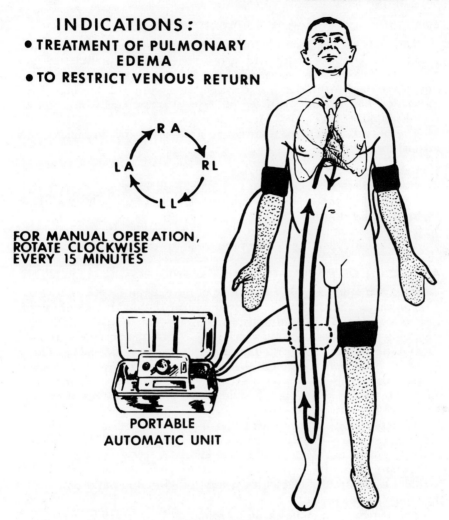

INDICATIONS:
- TREATMENT OF PULMONARY EDEMA
- TO RESTRICT VENOUS RETURN

FOR MANUAL OPERATION,
ROTATE CLOCKWISE
EVERY 15 MINUTES

PORTABLE
AUTOMATIC UNIT

FIG. 7–2. Rotating tourniquets.

a greater inflow of blood into the right ventricle and thereby increasing congestion. Morphine is given to decrease respirations, lessen dyspnea and reduce anxiety. In addition to a narcotic analgesic, a vasodilator is given as well as one of the newer intravenous diuretics such as Edecrine. The patient is rapidly digitalized to enhance myocardial contractions and control ventricular rate.

7. Cardiac rhythm should be watched carefully for arrhythmias.

APPLICATION OF AUTOMATIC ROTATING TOURNIQUETS

The cuffs of the rotating tourniquet are placed high on the four extremities. Pressure is adjusted above the diastolic pressure in each extremity. The cuffs are made tight enough to restrict venous return but not to interfere with arterial circulation. In Figure 7–2, the dotted cuff pattern on the patient's right leg indicates that the cuff is not inflated. Peripheral pulses are checked intermittently.

The automatic rotating tourniquet unit has many advantages over manual rotation:

1. It is more precise and dependable.
2. It affords immediate venostasis with relief to the patient.
3. It saves the time of doctors and nurses, who would otherwise rotate hand-applied tourniquets.
4. The cuffs are in place for evaluating the patient's blood pressure.
5. An automatic timer rotates the pressure in the cuff every 15 minutes.

APPLICATION OF MANUAL ROTATING TOURNIQUETS

The tourniquets are placed on three of the extremities at a time. Every 15 minutes, one tourniquet is removed and placed on the extremity that has no tourniquet. The tourniquets are always rotated in the same direction, either clockwise or counterclockwise. If rubber tourniquets are used, care must be taken not to cut off arterial circulation. If arterial circulation is cut off, permanent damage to the tissues may result. Frequent checking of the pulse on all extremities is necessary to assure adequate circulation. Blood pressure cuffs with an aneroid gauge permit inflation of the cuff just above the diastolic pressure.

An explanation to the patient that the rotating tourniquets will provide relief shortly will help lessen his anxiety, produced by the discomfort and the cyanotic discoloration of his extremities.

Pressure is always maintained in three cuffs. A rotating schedule occludes venous return of each extremity for 45 minutes at a time with a 15-minute release period.

The patient should be made as comfortable as possible during this procedure. If the treatment is to be continued for a long period, the skin should be protected from becoming too irritated. When the treatment is to be discontinued, one tourniquet is removed every 15 minutes. This permits a gradual increase in the amount of circulating blood that the heart and lungs must handle. To release all tourniquets at the same time would precipitate another attack of pulmonary edema.

Throughout the course of this treatment, assignment of one member of the team to the sole responsibility of the multiple duties is suggested.

Application of tourniquets is contraindicated:

1. If the patient is in shock or impending shock
2. If the patient has a peripheral embolus or ischemia of an extremity

To help reduce the cardiac load, the patient should be propped up high in bed or placed in a sitting position. This position plus gravity increase hydrostatic pressure in the veins and capillaries of the lower extremities. Fluid will then escape into the peripheral interstitial spaces, thereby reducing venous return.

RIGHT HEART FAILURE

Right heart failure usually follows left heart failure. Frequently the symptoms of right and left failure are combined and often appear simultaneously.

Signs of Failure

1. Cyanosis
2. Pleural effusion
3. Venous distention
4. Liver distention
5. Ascites
6. Oliguria
7. Edema

If pulmonary edema is present, cyanosis will be evident. The inability of the left ventricle to supply the arterial circulation causes engorgement of the pulmonary vessels. Serous fluid is therefore pushed into the pulmonary tissues, causing pulmonary edema and pleural effusion.

As right atrial pressure increases, resulting in increased capillary venous pressure, bulging jugular veins will be evident.

With reduced output from the right ventricle, failure is apparent in the splanchnic area and in the distal extremities. As venous pressure rises in the hepatic veins, the liver becomes congested and fluid escapes through the engorged capillary walls to form dependent edema and ascites.

With the reduced blood volume to the kidneys, the glomerular filtration rate is diminished, causing subsequent sodium and water retention in the interstitial space. Urinary output is scanty.

Edema formation is determined by elevated hydrostatic capillary pressure. In ambulatory patients, edema is localized in dependent parts of the body. In patients confined to bed, the edema localizes over the sacrum and back.

Treatment

The objectives in the management of congestive failure are:

1. To determine the factor responsible for its development
2. To improve cardiac efficiency
3. To control sodium–water retention.

Digitalis is valuable in treating congestive heart failure. It increases the force of systolic contractions and controls the ventricular rate.

Diuretics are given to promote the excretion of sodium and water. Daily intake and output records should be recorded.

Nursing Responsibilities

1. Be alert for early signs of congestive failure.
2. Examine the patient's back and legs for edema.
3. Observe neck veins for distention.
4. Keep an accurate intake and output record.

Bed rest is necessary to reduce the cardiac load. The failing heart cannot maintain an adequate output to meet the body's needs, and physical activity must therefore be kept at a minimum. Because of the increased incidence of arrhythmia in victims of heart failure, the patient is monitored. Premature beats and atrial fibrillation occur frequently.

Rest usually reduces the need for oxygen. Initially, oxygen may be given by catheter.

Fluid intake is usually restricted and a low sodium diet is ordered to control edema.

Other nursing measures include general hygienic measures with emphasis upon good care of the skin, passive leg exercises, and proper positioning in bed. The nurse should be alert for any signs of phlebothrombosis, a frequent complication.

VENOUS PRESSURE

An important diagnostic test used to confirm congestive heart failure is monitoring the central venous pressure.

Venous pressure is the pressure which blood exerts within the veins. It indicates the heart's ability to handle the returning venous blood. Venous pressure is elevated in congestive heart failure, hypervolemia and venous obstruction. External compression of the jugular vein increases venous pressure.

If venous pressure is to be measured over a period of time, a central venous pressure apparatus, involving the use of an intravenous catheter, is used.

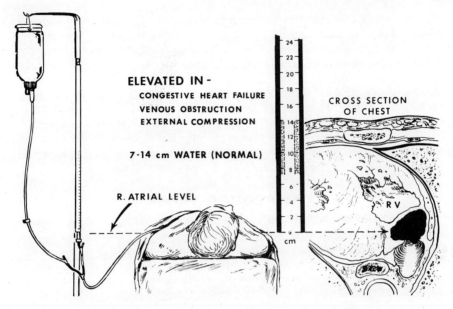

ELEVATED IN -
CONGESTIVE HEART FAILURE
VENOUS OBSTRUCTION
EXTERNAL COMPRESSION

7-14 cm WATER (NORMAL)

R. ATRIAL LEVEL

CROSS SECTION
OF CHEST

RV

cm

FIG. 7–3. Measuring central venous pressure.

There are several techniques for placement of a catheter in the central venous system:

1. Use a peripheral vein in the arm or leg.
2. Use a subclavian vein.
3. Use an external jugular vein.

After the catheter has been secured in the vein, it is connected to a disposable venous pressure set. Directions for attaching the set to a sterile solution of 5 per cent dextrose in water are included with the set.

Figure 7–3 shows the patient in a recumbent position so that his arm is supported at a level with his heart. After the catheter has been passed, the physician sets the level of the manometer scale and side arm tubing on the intravenous stand. The centimeter scale is taped to the stand with the zero mark on the scale at the right atrial level of the patient's heart.

The level of fluid in the manometer tubing will adjust to the patient's venous pressure. Normal venous pressure ranges from 7 to 14 cm. of water pressure.

Nursing Responsibilities

1. Explain test to patient.
2. Place patient in recumbent position if tolerated.
3. Assist physician.

The test is explained to the patient so that he will be psychologically prepared for it and will not experience undue anxiety. The patient should be in a comfortable position. If an antecubital vein is used, the patient's arm should be supported away from the body to avoid compression of the catheter as it curves in at the axillary line. If the patient is unable to lie flat, a satisfactory reading can be obtained if the head elevation is identical at each reading.

Presently, many physicians are using CVP (central venous pressure) as an aid in determining the amount of body-fluid replacement to avoid overloading the heart. This procedure is usually carried out at the patient's bedside by the physician with the assistance of the nurse.

CARDIOGENIC SHOCK

The shock associated with myocardial infarction usually appears abruptly. It is urgent that the treatment regimen be initiated promptly. The longer shock persists, the more intractable it becomes.

The causes of cardiogenic shock are not clear; however, it is associated with a great decrease in cardiac output resulting from the impairment of myocardial contractility.

Symptoms

1. Extreme weakness
2. Pallor
3. Cyanosis
4. Apathy
5. Dyspnea
6. Weak pulse
7. Hypotension
8. Sudden pulmonary edema
9. Congestive heart failure
10. Anuria

Due to a decreased supply of blood to the cells and skeletal muscles, the patient feels extremely weak.

The diminished cardiac output limits the amount of oxygenated blood to the skin, thereby causing ischemia. The skin becomes ashen gray with cyanosis of the lips and nail beds.

Lack of oxygen to the brain reduces its ability to function properly. The patient is not alert to what is happening to him and he appears indifferent, unable to respond emotionally. In this state the patient may require ventilatory assistance with a respirator, as shown in Figure 7–4.

Dyspnea associated with shock is due to pulmonary congestion. Heart contractions are rapid and very weak due to the weak left ventricle. The

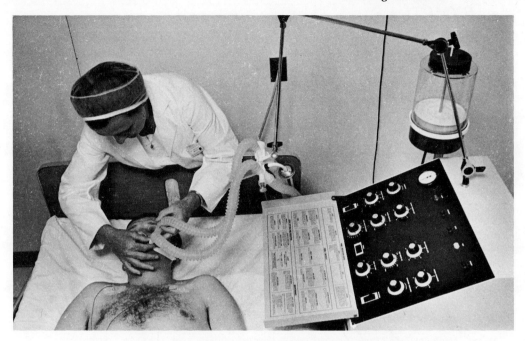

FIG. 7–4. Ventilation of patient with respirator.

rapid, severe reduction in cardiac output is responsible for the low blood pressure. With the reduction in cardiac output, the pulmonary capillaries become engorged and fluid then leaks into the alveoli.

Most patients with prolonged shock develop signs of congestive heart failure.

When cardiac output is less than normal, urinary output decreases. When cardiac output is reduced to one-half to two-thirds normal, renal function is so diminished that there is no urinary output.

Shock is sometimes irreversible. The patient may be in shock a number of days before he reaches the state where all therapeutic measures fail. In prolonged shock, there is a gradual loss of arterial tone and increasing myocardial depression. In this state death is imminent.

Treatment

Cardiogenic shock is one of the most difficult types of shock to treat. Preferred drugs, of course, are those which do not adversely affect the heart. Adrenergic vasopressors, which raise the systolic blood pressure and increase cardiac output, are currently used in the early course of shock.

Levarterenol and metaraminol are given intravenously. Careful obser-

SYMPTOMS

- COUGH
- SUDDEN PAIN
- TACHYCARDIA
- DROP IN BP
- RAPID RESPIRATIONS
- SUDDEN DYSPNEA
- MILD HEMOPTYSIS

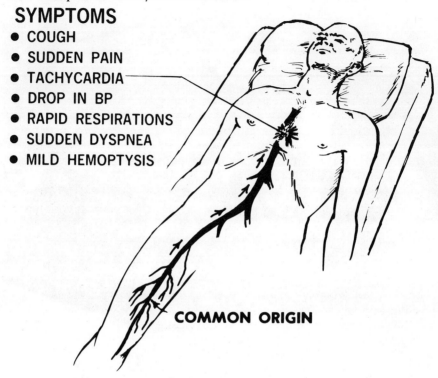

COMMON ORIGIN

Fig. 7–5. Pulmonary embolism.

vation is necessary to avoid excessive rises in blood pressure and the occurrence of cardiac arrhythmias.

Intravenous digitalis is given to strengthen cardiac contractions and to decrease the rate.

With increased cardiac output, glomerular filtration pressure is raised and the urinary output increases. Diuretics are then given to establish a balance between fluid intake and output.

An indwelling catheter is usually ordered to record an accurate hourly output. Increased output is a good indicator of diminishing renal ischemia.

Nursing Responsibilities

1. Prompt treatment is urgent to provide an adequate blood supply to the brain. Mental apathy is one of the earliest symptoms observed. The nurse must, therefore, be sensitive to the patient's mental status and alert the physician if mental apathy is observed.

2. The difference between the systolic and diastolic pressure is the pulse pressure. In shock there is a reduction in the pulse pressure. Frequent and accurate recordings of blood pressure are necessary to note a significant change.
3. Oxygen should be started immediately to help increase the oxygen content in the circulating blood. Oxygen given with a positive-pressure respirator assists in the alveolar expansion and diffusion of oxygen. Thus the hemoglobin in the pulmonary system becomes better saturated with oxygen.
4. Observe the cardiac rhythm frequently for the development of arrhythmias, which may occur with shock.
5. Emotional stress places an added burden on the incapacitated heart. Physical and emotional rest must be maintained if the patient is to recover.

PULMONARY EMBOLISM

Another complication of myocardial infarction is pulmonary embolism, shown in Figure 7–5, which may occur within 3 to 10 days of the attack. Venous stasis occurs with prolonged bed rest; blood flow is reduced and muscle tone is lost.

Most emboli originate from peripheral thrombi in the deep veins of the legs. Mural thrombi originate in the left ventricle or atrium.

Symptoms

1. Coughing
2. Cyanosis
3. Sudden chest pain
4. Tachycardia
5. Decreasing blood pressure
6. Rapid respiration
7. Sudden dyspnea
8. Mild hemoptysis

In addition to these, a sporadic cough is sometimes present.

The patient may experience sudden pain in either the right or left chest. This pain is aggravated by deep inspiration. If the embolism is significant, syncope, severe dyspnea and cyanosis may be the first symptoms.

Tachycardia is common and the patient complains of palpitations. The blood pressure drops and shock may soon follow. If the embolus is massive, the patient is restless and anxious, and may express a feeling of impending death.

The dyspnea with pulmonary embolus is severe; respiration is rapid and shallow.

Hemoptysis may be the first symptom. The blood is bright red, and in many patients it may be scanty.

Figure 7–5 demonstrates the origin of the thrombi in the deep veins of the lower extremities. All or part of a thrombus may break loose from its site and circulate. It may break up into smaller portions and pass through the right heart, occluding various branches of the pulmonary arterial tree.

If the pulmonary artery is occluded, blood flow ceases and death occurs suddenly.

LABORATORY FINDINGS

1. Leukocytosis
2. Elevated SLDH
3. Increased bilirubin

Treatment

Oxygen should be started promptly to relieve dyspnea.

Heparin is the drug of choice to prevent further clot formation. It may be given intravenously or subcutaneously for several weeks. Oral anticoagulants may then be used.

Start the treatment program for complications as they occur.

Nursing Responsibilities

1. Nursing care for the patient subject to prolonged bed rest should emphasize preventive nursing measures to prevent pooling of venous blood and aid circulation.
2. The substernal pain is similar to the pain of myocardial ischemia. Demerol or morphine is given to relieve pain and allay apprehension.
3. Passive arm and leg exercises should be done for 5 minutes at least 3 times a day.
4. Elastic stockings support the calves of the legs and prevent venous distention.
5. When anticoagulant therapy is started, the nurse must be alert for petechiae in the skin and for the presence of blood in the urine or stool.

CARDIAC ARREST

The possible causes of cardiac arrest are many. It may be diagnosed as cardiac standstill (asystole), in which the heartbeat is absent, ventricular fibrillation, in which the heartbeat is chaotic, or cardiovascular collapse, in which the heartbeat is rhythmic but ineffective.

When the cardiac arrest has been diagnosed, it is imperative that emergency heart–lung resuscitation be started immediately. Irreversible brain damage from anoxia occurs within 3 to 5 minutes.

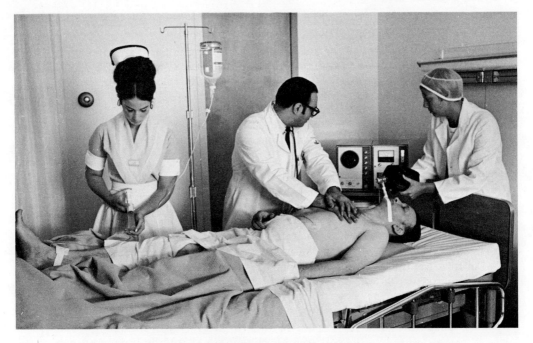

Fig. 7–6. Resuscitation.

Establishment of an Airway and Ventilation

Place the patient in a supine position on a firm, flat surface. Before resuscitation can begin, an open airway to the lungs must be established. In an unconscious person the jaw muscles relax and the tongue drops back to obstruct the airway. The best method to clear the airway is to:

1. Lift the neck with one hand.
2. Tilt the head back into maximum extension and clean out any fluids or objects in the oral cavity.

In many instances the patient will begin to breathe spontaneously as soon as the airway is opened.

If there is no evidence of breathing after the airway is opened, begin rhythmic lung inflation with mouth-to-mouth resuscitation. Close the nose to prevent the escape of air. Take a deep breath and place your mouth over the mouth of the patient. Make a tight seal and inflate his lungs until you see the chest rise. Allow the patient to exhale. Do this 3 to 5 times initially, then 12 times per minute.

If breathing is absent and there is no pulse after effective lung inflation, begin external cardiac compression (shown in Figure 7–6) in order to circulate the blood:

1. Place the heel of one hand over the lower half of the sternum and the heel of the other hand on top of the first.
2. Keep elbows straight and use the weight of the upper body to exert 60 to 100 pounds of pressure vertically to depress the sternum 1½ to 2 inches. This compresses the heart between the sternum and the vertebrae and forces the blood to circulate.
3. At the end of each stroke, the hands are relaxed to enable full chest expansion and permit the heart to fill with blood.
4. Sternal compression is repeated once every second. The patient should be ventilated 2 or 3 times per 10 to 15 sternal compressions.

During resuscitation, the femoral or carotid pulse should be checked frequently to determine effective circulation. Also the pupils should be checked for constriction. Dilation of the pupils is an ominous sign.

Resuscitation measures should be continued as long as the patient responds or if there is evidence of cardiac activity on the ECG strip.

An automatic heart–lung resuscitator should be used if it is available, since it ventilates the lungs and circulates blood more uniformly than manual resuscitation, thereby increasing the patient's chances of survival.

Nursing Responsibilities in Asystole

1. When cardiac arrest occurs in the coronary care unit, the low-rate alarm on the cardioscope sounds. The event should be timed and confirmed with a continuous ECG tracing.
2. Sound the physician alarm.
3. A sharp, hard blow to the precordium may restore the heartbeat.
4. Start the automatic timer set for 2 minutes. Resuscitation must begin before cerebral anoxia occurs.
5. Do not wait for the physician. Start the external pacemaker if it has not been set on the automatic position to start when the low-rate alarm sounds.
6. If external pacing fails, start pulmonary and cardiac resuscitation within 2 minutes.
7. If cardiac arrest is due to ventricular fibrillation, the treatment is electrical defibrillation as described in Chapter 5.

The following drugs should be available:

1. Sodium bicarbonate, which may be given within 5 minutes to combat acidosis and improve cerebral flow
2. Epinephrine to improve blood pressure and cardiac tone
3. Calcium gluconate to increase cardiac output
4. Quinidine to decrease myocardial irritability

5. Isuprel to stimulate forceful ventricular contractions
6. Levophed to maintain blood pressure
7. Pronestyl or lidocaine to combat fibrillation

VENTRICULAR RUPTURE

After occlusion of one of the coronary arteries or its branches, scar tissue begins to form at the edges of the damaged area. A mild scar appears within 6 to 10 days.

Most deaths from myocardial infarction occur within the first week, resulting from an irreversible arrhythmia. However, a small percentage of patients die from rupture of the ventricle. Death due to ventricular rupture is sudden. The rupture leads to hemopericardium, and the patient dies of cardiac tamponade. Most ventricular ruptures occur about the fourth or fifth day following infarction, at the infarction site where it joins healthy tissue. The complication is more common in women than in men, and occurs only in transmural infarctions.

Less common are rupture of the ventricular septum or rupture of papillary muscle. In these types of ruptures, death is not so sudden, but the prognosis is extremely poor.

Healing of the infarcted area occurs with scar tissue replacing the destroyed muscle, which does not regenerate. Necrosis of muscle and leukocyte infiltration occur in the first week. Necrotic muscle is replaced by connective tissue in the second week.

After the first week, the patient may feel well and want to resume his normal activities. In order for the myocardium to repair itself by scar-tissue formation and to establish collateral circulation to the injured area, physical activity must be limited.

Complete bed rest is indicated for several weeks, followed by a planned program of increased activity. At the end of 2 months, tough scar-tissue formation enables the patient to resume most normal activities.

Other complications which may occur include:

1. Cerebral emboli may originate in the left ventricular mural thrombi, resulting in a cerebral vascular accident.
2. Peripheral emboli, which originate in the left ventricular mural thrombi, usually lodge at the bifurcation of the femoral or common iliac arteries.
3. Pericarditis, which may occur 2 to 5 days after myocardial infarction, usually disappears spontaneously. In the presence of a pericardial rub, anticoagulants may be discontinued due to the possibility of cardiac tamponade.

REFERENCES AND BIBLIOGRAPHY

Beland, I.: Clinical Nursing. pp. 561-731. New York, Macmillan, 1965.

Brunner, L. S., Emerson, C. P., Ferguson, L. K., and Suddarth, D. S.: Textbook of Medical-Surgical Nursing. ed. 2. pp. 359-392. Philadelphia, J. B. Lippincott, 1970.

Cooper, T., and Dempsey, R.: Assisted circulation. I. Mod. Conc. Cardiov. Dis., 37:95-100, (May) 1968.

Friedberg, C. K.: Diseases of the Heart. ed. 3. pp. 219-242, 284-304, 443-474, 483-575, 583-628, 643-693, 676-678, 706-763, 770-791, 866-922. Philadelphia, W. B. Saunders, 1966.

Guyton, A. C.: Textbook of Medical Physiology. ed. 3. pp. 179-194, 233-243, 301-310, 312-320, 371-382. Philadelphia, W. B. Saunders, 1966.

Hanchett, E. S., and Johnson, R. A.: Early signs of congestive heart failure. Am. J. Nurs., 68:1456-1461, (July) 1968.

Hurst, J. W., and Logue, R. R.: The Heart. pp. 224-234, 239-282, 285-341, 350-362. New York, McGraw-Hill, 1966.

Lown, B.: Intensive heart care. Sci. Am., 219:19-27, (July) 1968.

MacBryde, C.: Signs and Symptoms. ed. 4. pp. 262-308, 335. Philadelphia, J. B. Lippincott, 1964.

Meltzer, L. E., et al.: Intensive Coronary Care—A Manual for Nurses. CCU Fund, Philadelphia Presbyterian Hospital, 1965.

Minogue, W. F., Smessart, A. A., and Grace, W. J.: External cardiac massage for cardiac arrest due to myocardial infarction. Am. J. Cardiol., 13:25-29, (Jan.) 1964.

Nachlas, M. M., and Miller, D. J.: Closed chest cardiac resuscitation in patients with acute myocardial infarction. Am. Heart J., 69:448-459, (April) 1965.

Nett, M., and Petty, T.: Acute respiratory failure. Am. J. Nurs., 67:1847-1853, (Sept.) 1967.

Rodman, M., and Smith, D.: Pharmacology and Drug Therapy in Nursing. pp. 275-368. Philadelphia, J. B. Lippincott, 1968.

Sasahara, A., and Foster, V.: Pulmonary embolism. Am. J. Nurs., 67:1634-1641, (Aug.) 1967.

Shafer, K. N., Sawyer, J. R., McClusky, A. M., and Beck, E. L.: Medical-Surgical Nursing. ed. 4. pp. 317-346, 358-361. St. Louis, C. V. Mosby, 1967.

Smith, D. W., and Gips, C. D.: Care of the Adult Patient. ed. 2. pp. 529-580, 627-637. Philadelphia, J. B. Lippincott, 1966.

Wood, P.: Diseases of the Heart and Circulation. ed. 3. Philadelphia, J. B. Lippincott, 1968.

8 ELECTRICAL BASIS OF CARDIAC MONITORING

The heart beats and functions as the pump of the circulatory system in response to its own self-generated electrical impulses.

The nurse who is charged with the responsibility of cardiac monitoring must have some understanding of:

1. How this electrical activity originates
2. How the electrocardiograph transcribes this activity into graphs
3. Normal pathways of electrical stimulation of the heart
4. Abnormal pathways, their cause and significance
5. Relationship of monitor findings to clinical findings
6. Accepted forms of treatment of abnormalities and their underlying rationale
7. Recognition of those emergencies in which the medical staff of the hospital authorizes the nurse to initiate specific treatment under written policy and procedure

ELECTRICITY

Researchers into the phenomenon of the beating heart work in many disciplines: physics, chemistry, electrochemistry, anatomy, physiology, and so on. The nurse must know basic scientific concepts from many fields in order to understand the principles of cardiac monitoring. A review of vocabulary and major principles underlying monitoring follows:

Force is that which produces or prevents motion or has a tendency to do so.

Motion is a continuing change of place or position.

Work is the product of motion and force.

Resistance is the opposition of one force to another.

Energy is the capacity to do work. There are two kinds of energy: **kinetic energy** and **potential energy.** Kinetic energy results from the motion of a mass, such as a rolling ball, a moving car. Potential energy is stored energy, such as a parked car. Matter and energy are interchangeable ($E=MC^2$); they cannot be created or destroyed, but only converted from one form to another. There are many forms of energy—heat, mechanical, magnetic, electrical, chemical, light, sound, and atomic or nuclear.

A **charge** is potential electrical energy, which may be positive or negative. It is a latent electrical force which exists because of the nearness of one electrified body to another. A **current** is electrical charge in motion.

The **atom** is the smallest particle of an element that can exist either by itself or in combination with other atoms. It has a dense central core called the nucleus, which is composed of **protons** and (except for protium, an isotopic form of hydrogen) **neutrons.** Protons carry a positive electrical charge; neutrons carry no charge. Electrons, which carry a negative charge, move around the nucleus in orbitals, groups of which are called energy levels or shells. The aggregate of electrons forms what is called the electron cloud. Whereas protons and electrons are charged, atoms are electrically neutral; they must therefore contain equal numbers of protons and electrons. The number and arrangement of the protons and electrons account for the chemical properties of the atom.

Elements are substances which cannot be broken down into simpler substances by ordinary means, for example iron, oxygen and silver. The atoms of any one element differ from the atoms of other elements.

Certain atoms are temporarily able to hold more than their normal number of electrons. When two different substances such as glass and silk are put into good contact by being rubbed together, some electrons leave the glass and attach themselves to the silk. The glass now has a deficiency of negative charge, which means it is positively charged in relationship to the silk, which has taken on additional negativity.

Like charges repel each other, while unlike charges attract. An electrical charge will tend to move from one place to another if electrical potential difference exists. We have all seen the electric spark "created" when Nylon uniforms are subjected to friction by the motion of the wearer.

Conductors. Those substances which allow electrons to pass easily are called *conductors.* If it is to keep its charge, a charged body must be surrounded by something that does not allow electrons to pass freely. In other words, the presence of some form of resistance is required.

In an electric lamp cord, the metal wire is conductive and the current can pass freely along it. The protective covering is resistant, or non-conductive. The charge cannot pass through it. If the protective covering is broken, the electric current can seek the path of least resistance to the nearest, most conductive material. Because of its chemical content, the human body is an excellent conductor, as many can testify who have received a "shock" from a defective or ungrounded appliance.

Ions and electrolytes. An ion is an atom or group of atoms, which, by either gaining or losing one or more electrons, forms particles with unbalanced electrostatic charges. A negatively charged particle (anion) is an atom which has gained one or more electrons. A positively charged particle (cation) is an atom which has lost one or more electrons. Substances that conduct electricity by means of ions are called *electrolytes*. Acids, bases and salts are electrolytes.

Knowledge of the characteristics of electricity has made it possible to harness this energy by the use of the generator, which changes mechanical energy into electrical energy. Applying the principles of conduction and resistance, current can be sent along specific pathways to end points: to the radio, to be converted to sound; to the light bulb, to be converted to light; to the heater, to be converted to heat; to the television screen, to be converted to wave patterns which present pictures in motion.

Magnetism is sometimes called the "electrical twin." It is the property of attracting iron, probably due to electron motion in the atom. It is theorized that, due to strong electric currents in huge mineral deposits in the core of the earth, the earth itself acts as a large magnet, with one pole of the magnet north, and one pole south.

The ordinary compass needle is a bar magnet. The end of the compass needle attracted to the earth's south pole is called the south-seeking pole. The end of the compass needle attracted to the earth's north pole is called the north-seeking pole. Polarity is described as the condition of being positively or negatively charged in relationship to a magnetic pole.

A compass needle placed just below a current-carrying wire takes up a position perpendicular to the wire while the current is flowing through. If the direction of current flow is reversed, the angle of the needle is still perpendicular, but the needle ends are reversed. In other words, an electric current produces a magnetic field in its neighborhood. Currents in solution give the same effect.

The **galvanometer** is an instrument for detecting and determining the direction and force of flow of electric current. Using the principle of the compass needle, the direction of deflection is based on polarity; the degree of deflection is based on the strength of current.

ELECTROPHYSIOLOGY

Every living thing is composed of protoplasm, a jelly-like fluid material. Protoplasm is extremely complex chemically. It contains hydrogen, chlorine, nitrogen, sodium, calcium, potassium, magnesium and other elements.

The cell is the smallest unit of living matter. It consists of a mass of protoplasm, usually enclosed in a thin membrane wall. Inside the cell is denser protoplasm, called the nucleus. The protoplasm outside the nucleus is called cytoplasm.

In the watery solution of the cell certain atoms form ions which, as we have seen, are electrically charged particles. Solutions containing ions conduct electrical current.

The electrical potential exists in the cell due to its chemical make-up. The electrical impulse that starts the heartbeat and the beat itself depend on a balanced ratio of sodium, potassium, calcium, oxygen and some form of energy-producing glucose.

Both sodium and potassium carry positive charges, but there are many more sodium ions than potassium ions in the extracellular fluid. Furthermore, the positively charged potassium ions within the cell are outnumbered by the positively charged sodium ions outside the cell. Thus, the outside of the cell is more positive than the inside. The inside of the cell is negative in relation to the outside. The membrane potential is about —90 millivolts. This means that negativity on the inside of the membrane is 90 millivolts greater than on the outside. (A millivolt is 1/1000 of a volt. It takes a 9-volt battery to operate the ordinary portable transistor radio.)

The passage of sodium ions through the cell membrane to the exterior of the cell is effected by a transport mechanism known as the "sodium pump." This is a complicated process, involving the permeability of the cell membrane as well as the size and weight of the ions, and, of course, the whole action of cellular metabolism governs the concentration gradients of sodium across the cell membrane. Since the process of the sodium pump leads to a high concentration of postive sodium ions, with a consequent positivity on the outside of the membrane opposed by a negativity on the inside, it is primarily this mechanism that produces the normal electrical gradient across the cell membrane. The tendency of the positively charged sodium ions to attract negative particles from within the cell has much to do with controlling the size of the cell and with the prevention of its swelling and even bursting. Thus, at least indirectly, the sodium pump exerts some effect on the pressure gradient across the cell membrane.

The high concentration of potassium ions within the cell seems to depend not only on the transport mechanism, but also upon the membrane potential which is caused by the sodium pump.

It is as if the individual cell were a small charged battery, the strength of the charge equaling the electrical potential difference between the inside and the outside of the cell.

At this point, stimulation of the cell membrane results in many sodium ions pouring into the cell and a few potassium ions escaping from the cell. The inside of the cell is now relatively positive.

An electrical potential difference now exists between this cell and its neighbor, and a current discharges between the two. Successive stimulation from cell to cell perpetuates this "action current," which we now speak of as "propagation of impulse" or "depolarization wave." The advantage of this chain-like reaction is that the electrical force is not reduced before it reaches muscle-contracting fibers, as each cell is stimulated by its neighbor with precisely the same voltage.

This biologic electric current relays the impulse over conducting tissue, from cell to cell, to the muscle-contracting fibers, where it triggers the breakdown of ATP (adenosine triphosphate), which releases chemical energy for muscle contraction.

After releasing its potential, each cell then allows sodium to be pushed out of the cell and potassium to flow back in. The cell "battery" has been recharged and is ready to discharge again.

In its resting state, the cell is said to be **polarized**; in its discharging state, **depolarized**; and in its return to rest, **repolarized**.

In atrial and ventricular muscle fibers, the cellular transmembrane potential characteristically remains constant during diastole, at approximately 90 mv. Upon stimulation, rapid depolarization occurs, followed by a return to normal resting potential.

Automaticity

Automaticity is that property of heart cells which enable them to initiate spontaneously their own rhythmic cardiac excitation impulse, without the intervention of external agencies. In diastole, cells which possess automaticity exhibit a slow depolarization process which continues until the transmembrane potential falls to approximately 40 mv. This is followed by rapid depolarization which propagates an impulse which is conducted over the heart. Then the transmembrane potential returns to the resting potential of approximately —90 mv.

Automaticity is characteristic of many heart cells. These automatic cells generate and discharge impulses at a rate specific to the area from which they derive. The intrinsic automatic rate of the cell is determined by the speed of slow depolarization to the threshold value of 40 mv. when rapid depolarization takes over. Cells which demonstrate automaticity are located in:

1. The S-A (sino-atrial) node—a primary pacemaker with an automatic rate of approximately 60–100 impulses per minute
2. The junctional area—a secondary pacemaker with an automatic rate of approximately 40–60 impulses per minute
   a. The A-N (atrial-nodal) section
   b. The N (node) section
   c. The N-H (nodal-His) section

3. The bundle branches
4. The peripheral Purkinje fibers—a tertiary pacemaker with an automatic rate of approximately 20–40 impulses per minute

Pacemakers

The cell or group of cells that generates and discharges at the fastest rate ordinarily takes over the role of *pacemaker,* because the excitation wave it initiates extinguishes any immature impulse formation in other areas by depolarization.

The automatic rates of pacemaking fibers can be markedly changed by both physiological and pathological states. Intrinsic pacemaker rates can be slowed down or speeded up by metabolic demand and by regulation from the central nervous system.

Conduction System

Normally the electrical impulse for cardiac contraction originates in the S-A node. It was formerly believed that there were no specialized conducting fibers within the atria or from one atrium to the other, and that the electrical impulse was propagated from muscle cell to muscle cell, each cell stimulating its neighbor.

Because the impulse arising in the S-A node reaches the A-V node faster than would be possible if conduction were as described above, it is now generally agreed that special conduction pathways do exist, but it is not yet generally agreed where they are or what their function is in the human heart.

The excitation wave is slowed down by decreased conductivity as it reaches the junctional area. It passes on through the common bundle, to the left and right bundle branches, and to the network-like structure of the Purkinje fibers. This portion of the electrical cycle is extremely fast since the electrical impulse is passing along highly conductive fibers.

The electrical activity recorded by the electrocardiogram precedes muscular response. It is not the equivalent of, nor does it follow, muscular contraction.

Stimulus–Response Cycle

While the myriad muscle cells are stimulated at infinitesimally small time differences, the muscles composed of these cells respond as a unit.

The impulse arising in the S-A node spreads out over the atria, and the atrial muscles contract. It travels over the specialized conductive tissue to the ventricular muscle cells, and the ventricular muscles contract.

REPOLARIZATION

As each cell discharges (depolarizes), it immediately starts to recharge (repolarize). The cell that depolarizes first repolarizes first, but repolarization proceeds at a slower rate than depolarization. At all times, then, in the living heart, some cells are depolarized, some are repolarizing, and some are repolarized.

REFRACTORY PERIOD

An important feature of the stimulus–response cycle is the refractory period. This period is divided as follows:

1. **Absolute.** The period in which no stimulus can evoke a response (the greater part of the contraction period), because the electrical changes which brought about the contraction are now being reversed, and preparation is being made for another stimulus–response cycle. This is a protective mechanism to heart muscle since it prevents the muscle from responding to all the impulses of extremely rapid pacemakers. Conceivably, responding to each impulse of excessively rapid pacemakers could throw the heart muscle into a state of tetanic contraction.
2. **Relative.** The period of repolarization in which a response can be elicited by a stimulus. During this period, the repolarization process is almost, but not quite, complete. Conduction can occur, but at a slower than normal rate. However, if a stimulus should occur often enough and fast enough in the relative refractory period, a serious problem of arrhythmia could occur.

The duration of the refractory period is not the same in all heart cells. It is shortest in atrial cells, longer in ventricular cells, and still longer in A-V nodal tissue. The duration of the refractory period varies with the heart rate. It also changes in response to some medications and to electrolyte disturbances.

The Atrio-Ventricular Junction

The electrical activity of the A-V node and bundle of His is not seen in the body surface electrocardiogram. The determination of normal or abnormal conduction through this area has been arrived at by deduction from effects seen in other portions of the ECG recording. The direct recording of electrical potentials by the placement of micro-electrodes has corroborated some of these deductions and brought about some changes in thinking about impulse generation and conduction. Such intracellular recordings have also given information on conduction velocity. The faster the rate of rise and the greater the amplitude of action current, the faster the conduction velocity.

The A-V node is divided functionally into three sections. What was formerly called *upper nodal* is now referred to as the A-N or atrial section, in which there are pacemaker fibers; *middle nodal* is now referred to as the N section, in which there are probably no pacemaker fibers;

lower nodal is now referred to as the N-H (for His) section, in which there are pacemaker fibers.

The A-V node is activated early during the P wave of the surface ECG. The main delay in A-V transmission occurs in the atrial margin of the node. Conduction then progressively increases in velocity within the node and bundle, down to the Purkinje fibers.

It must be remembered that the conductive system is capable of conducting in two directions. When it follows normal pathways from atria to ventricles, it is called orthograde conduction. When the conduction is backward from ventricles to atria, it is called retrograde conduction.

In retrograde conduction the same relative speeds hold true, except that retrograde conduction at the atrial margin is even slower than orthograde.

CONDUCTION BLOCK

Failure to permit the passage of electrical impulse along a conduction pathway is called "conduction block." Most disturbances of atrioventricular conduction occur at the A-V junction. However, bilateral blocking in the bundle branches prevents conduction from atria to ventricles as effectively as a block in the A-V node itself.

Potassium Effects on Excitation

The integrity of the stimulus–response cycle depends upon balanced ratios of sodium, potassium, calcium oxygen and some form of glucose.

Hypokalemia (serum potassium deficiency) increases resting membrane potential and reduces membrane excitability. The speed of exit of potassium from the cell is increased. It potentiates the effect of digitalis, and may result in atrial and ventricular arrhythmias because of increased irritability of the myocardium. Normal serum potassium level is 3.8 to 5.5 mEq. per liter. Adverse effects may appear at 3.0 mEq.[1]

Hyperkalemia (excess of serum potassium) decreases resting membrane potential and reduces intensity of action potential by slowing the exit of potassium from the cell. It slows impulse formation and conduction, slows heart rate, and produces blocks and standstill. Definite slowing of conduction occurs at 7 to 9 mEq. per liter.[2] At levels of 9 mEq. and above, pacemaker blocks may occur, thereby allowing the development of serious arrhythmias, atrial standstill or cardiac arrest.

---

[1] Corday, E., and Irving, D. W.: Disturbances of Heart Rate, Rhythm and Conduction. ed. 2. p. 269. Philadelphia, W. B. Saunders, 1962.

[2] *Op. cit.,* pp. 266-268.

ECG Changes in Electrolyte Disturbances

There are no absolutely diagnostic ECG changes due to any of the electrolyte imbalances. Specific changes in pattern are often associated with certain electrolyte disorders, but because these changes also occur in myocardial infarction, laboratory confirmation of serum electrolyte levels is needed. Changes due to electrolyte problems usually appear in all leads, as opposed to the more localized changes of myocardial infarction.

Hypercalcemia is manifested in the ECG by premature atrial and ventricular beats, due to increased myocardial irritability. The Q-T interval is shortened.

Hypocalcemia is manifested by prolonged Q-T interval, prolonged S-T segment, and normal T waves as shown in Figure 8–1.

Hypokalemia, or low serum potassium, increases cell membrane potential and decreases cell membrane permeability, producing increased myocardial irritability. It is manifested in the ECG by T wave flattening, S-T depression, preterminal T wave inversion and heightening of the U wave as shown in Figure 8–2. Associated with hypokalemia are premature atrial and ventricular beats, nodal tachycardia, atrial fibrillation, and atrial tachycardia with A-V block.

Hyperkalemia, or elevated serum potassium, decreases cell membrane potential and increases cell membrane permeability, thus predisposing to disturbances of conduction.

The T wave becomes tall, symmetrical and tent-shaped. There is S-T depression, the U wave disappears, the P wave flattens and both the

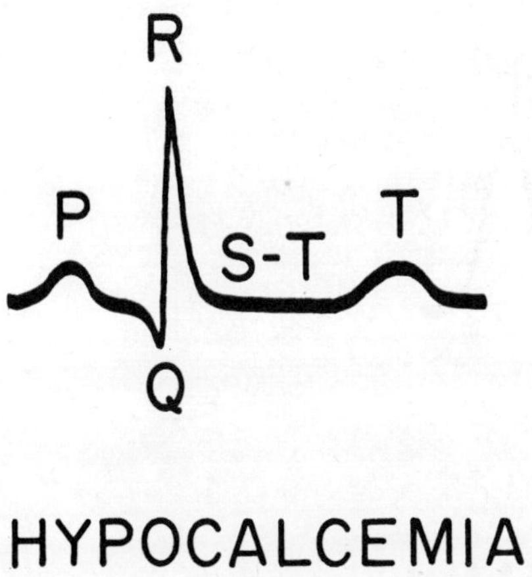

HYPOCALCEMIA

FIGURE 8–1

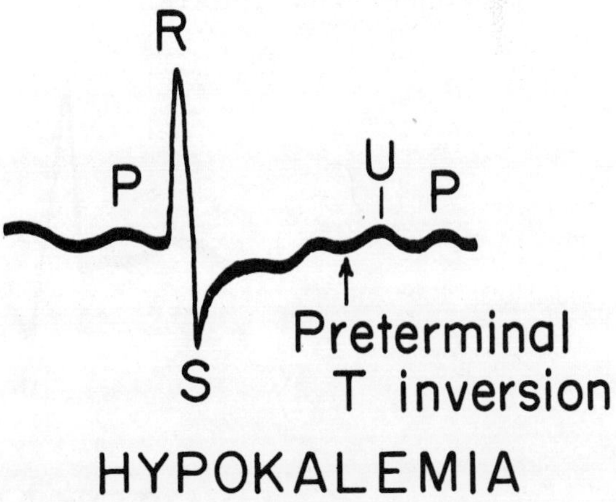

HYPOKALEMIA

FIGURE 8–2

P-R and QRS intervals prolong as shown in Figure 8–3. Associated with hyperkalemia are premature ventricular beats, ventricular flutter, idioventricular rhythm, ventricular fibrillation, atrial standstill, A-V block and cardiac arrest.

THE CARDIO-REGULATORY SYSTEM

The nerve supply to the heart is primarily concerned with the functions of pacemaking and conduction. The nervous control is both sympathetic (accelerator) and parasympathetic (inhibitor).

SYMPATHETIC

The sympathetic nervous system in the medulla sends fibers from the cervical ganglia via the cardiac nerves to the S-A node, atrial muscle, A-V node and ventricular muscle. Norepinephrine is released at the nerve endings. Norepinephrine increases the permeability of cell membrane to sodium. The altered sodium concentration in the cell results in increased excitability and shortened refractory period, with the following effects:

1. S-A node—increased rate of impulse formation
2. Atrial muscle—increased force of contraction
3. A-V node—increased speed of conduction
4. Ventricular muscle—increased force of contraction

PARASYMPATHETIC (VAGAL)

The parasympathetic nervous system sends fibers from the medulla via the vagus nerves to the S-A node, atrial muscle, A-V node, upper portion of bundle and the coronary vessels. There is believed to be no vagal nerve supply to the ventricles.

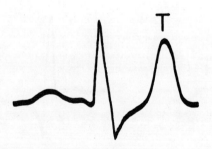

HYPERKALEMIA

FIGURE 8–3

Acetylcholine is released at the nerve endings. Acetylcholine increases the permeability of cell membrane to potassium. The altered potassium concentration in the cells results in decreased excitability and lengthened refractory period, with the following effects:

1. S-A node—decreased rate of impulse formation. Strong vagal stimulation can stop impulse formation
2. Atrial muscle—decreased force of contraction
3. A-V node—slows conduction rate and can cause varying degrees of block. Strong vagal stimulation can stop A-V conduction. The cardiac slowing results in greater diastolic filling and larger stroke volume.

SYMPATHETIC VASOCONSTRICTOR CENTER

The sympathetic vasoconstrictor center in the medulla sends nerve fibers to the blood vessels. There, special receptor nerve endings cause constriction of peripheral arteries and consequent elevation of blood pressure.

FEEDBACK TO CARDIO-REGULATORY SYSTEM

The following are factors which achieve their effect by influencing the central nervous system:

1. **Acidosis** (arterial pH under 7.4) stimulates the cardio-accelerator and vasoconstrictor centers, overriding vagal influence and thus increasing heart rate.
2. **Alkalosis** (arterial pH over 7.4) stimulates vagus and slows pulse rate.
3. **Elevated blood pressure** in the aorta or carotid sinus sends impulse to vagus, which results in cardiac slowing and vasodilation.
4. **Drop in blood pressure** in aorta or carotid sinus sends impulse to vasoconstrictor center and cardio-accelerator, which results in vasoconstriction and cardiac acceleration.
5. **Increased pressure** in pulmonary veins, vena cava or right atrium sends impulse to cardiac accelerator, which results in increased heart rate.
6. **Lungs** have nerve endings which send impulses via the vagus to the cardio-regulatory center. Inspiration inhibits vagus and increases heart rate. Expiration stimulates vagus and slows heart rate.
7. **Overt anxiety** may affect the hypothalamus or the vagal center. The former results in tachycardia or hypertension, the latter in bradycardia and hypotension.

THE ELECTROCARDIOGRAPH AND OSCILLOSCOPE

The human body is an excellent conductor. The electrical forces at work in the initiation of the heartbeat transmit themselves outward to the body surface. A suitable instrument, embodying the principles of the compass needle and the galvanometer, makes it possible to record the direction and strength of these electrical forces. The suitable instrument is, of course, the electrocardiograph and its companion, the oscilloscope.

The objective of the electrocardiogram is to record the action current of the heart on a time basis. The word "current" is here used very loosely. Current implies flow in a direct path. What we actually have in the millions of heart cells is a constantly changing polarity of one cell in relation to its neighbors in many directions. While we think of the electrical activation wave as being a single directional force, it is actually a result of forces in many directions.

A **vector** is a quantity, such as force or velocity, having direction and magnitude. The addition of vectors is a resultant force, for example:

1. A rope with a man and a woman pulling eastward at the same end of the rope. The man pulls with a force of 100 lbs., the woman with a force of 30 lbs. The resultant force is 130 lbs. east.
2. A rope with a man and a woman pulling at opposite ends. The man is pulling east with 100 lbs. of force. The woman is pulling west with 30 lbs. of force. The resultant force is 70 lbs. east.

An **electrode** is either of the two terminals of an electric source, the anode being positive and the cathode being negative. By placing a positive electrode and a negative electrode on the body surface, we parallel the situation of the current-carrying wire and compass needle.

The amount of current discharged by the body cell is so small that it must be amplified electronically to be recordable. An approaching depolarization wave produces a positive potential at the recording electrode. A receding wave of depolarization produces a negative potential at the recording electrode. The ECG graph, then, is a continuing recording of the electrical potential difference between the positive and negative electrodes. A **wave** pattern is the resultant recording. It can be recorded as a direct write-out, in which a heated stylus burns a pattern on the wax ECG paper. It can be visualized on a continuing basis on a television-type screen, the oscilloscope.

The ECG machine and oscilloscope are so designed that when there is no electrical potential difference between the positive and negative electrode, a flat line is recorded—the iso-electric line. When electrical potential difference exists, the base line becomes a series of undulations, with deflections above and below the iso-electric line. The deflections above the line result from the depolarization wave flowing toward the positive electrode. The deflections below the line result from the depolarization wave receding from the positive electrode. The dimensions of the wave pattern are determined by the distance of the recording electrode from depolarizing muscle, the mass of muscle being depolarized, the nature of the medium separating the current source from the recording electrode, and the rate of flow of the action current.

The pathway between a positive electrode and a negative electrode is called a **lead.** The total electrocardiogram is a recording of the electrical activity in many leads. Just as a piece of sculpture can tell us more than a two-dimensional photograph, multiple photographs can tell us more than a single photograph. Norms have been established for the wave patterns in all leads, and the use of multiple leads facilitates anatomical localization.

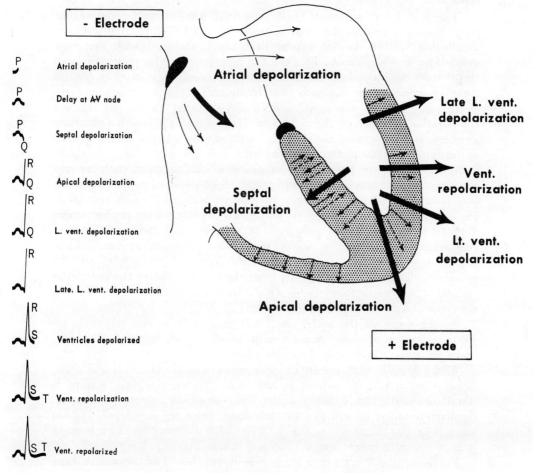

FIG. 8–4. Depolarization-repolarization in lead II.

Variations within the norm occur due to positional variation of the heart within the chest cavity. These variations are known as **axis deviations**. Axis changes are recognizable in the total ECG, and it is important for the physician to distinguish them from the changes due to ventricular enlargement.

In the many leads taken in the full electrocardiogram, the positive electrode is variably placed. The ECG records a positive deflection when current is flowing toward the positive electrode. A wave that is normally positive in one lead can therefore be normally negative in another.

LEAD II

The lead most commonly used in cardiac monitoring is lead II, because it usually records the most voltage and a tall P wave. If P waves of satisfactory voltage do not appear in lead II, the lead with the most satisfactory P wave should be used for monitoring. The relationship of the P wave to the other waves and complexes of the electrical cardiac cycle is essential in the diagnosis of arrhythmia.

In using lead II, the positive electrode is placed on the left leg and the negative electrode on the right arm. If we regard the positive electrode as an eye looking toward the negative electrode, lead II is looking upward at the diaphragmatic surface of the heart.

With the help of Figure 8–4, let us follow the electrical pathway and wave pattern of a single heartbeat in lead II. In depolarization, potassium leaves the cell and sodium enters. In repolarization, potassium returns to the cell and sodium leaves. In the atria, repolarization begins where depolarization begins, but progresses at a slower rate, hence the smaller repolarization waves. The waves of atrial repolarization are hidden. Septal depolarization normally proceeds from left to right. In the ventricles, depolarization proceeds from the endocardial to the epicardial surface. The apex depolarizes before the base. Repolarization occurs from the epicardial to the endocardial surface.

At the onset of the cycle, the heart muscle is at rest—there is no electrical potential difference between positive and negative electrode, and a short, flat, iso-electric line is inscribed.

The S-A node initiates an impulse which spreads out over the atria. Because the S-A node is high in the right atrium, the right atrium is stimulated first. The P wave is the first wave and it represents atrial depolarization. It is upright in deflection, because the depolarization wave is in the direction of the positive left-leg electrode. The P wave is up to 3 mm. in height, and 0.11 second in duration.

Following the P wave is a short iso-electric line. This represents slow

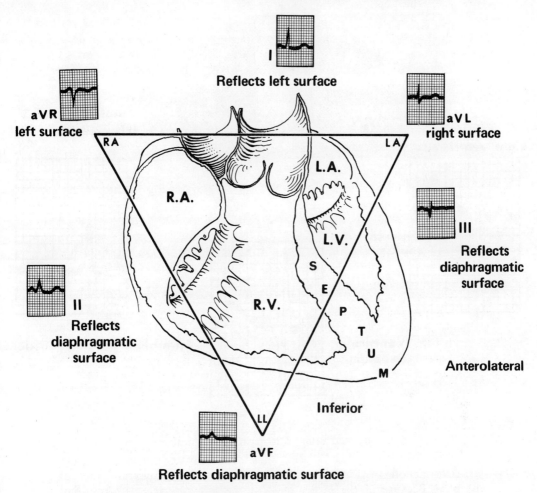

Reflects left surface

aVR
left surface

aVL
right surface

L.A.

R.A.

RA

LA

L.V.

III

**Reflects
diaphragmatic
surface**

S
E
R.V.   P
T
U
M

II

**Reflects
diaphragmatic
surface**

Anterolateral

Inferior

LL

aVF

Reflects diaphragmatic surface

Fig. 8–5. Normal ECG patterns in bipolar and augmented leads.

conduction through the A-V node, but so few cells are being depolarized that the ECG cannot pick up the electrical potential differences.

The Q wave is the first negative deflection. It is very small, less than 0.04 second in duration, and represents septal depolarization, which normally takes place from left to right—away from the positive electrode on the left leg.

The depolarization wave now travels rapidly through the common bundle, right and left bundle branches, and Purkinje fibers. Both

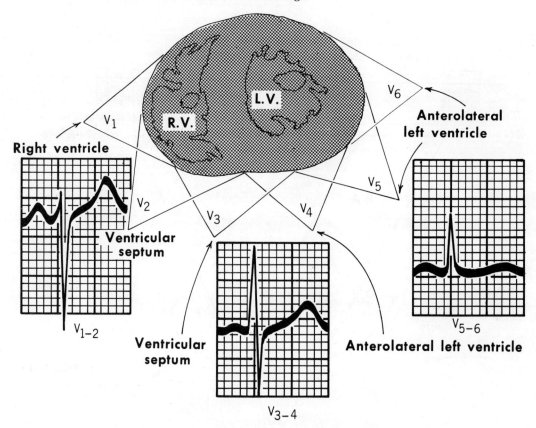

FIG. 8–6. Normal ECG patterns in V leads.

ventricles depolarize almost simultaneously, first at the apex and then at the base. Because of the larger mass of the left ventricle, the resultant electrical force is predominantly toward the left. This gives rise to the tall, upright R wave. As the ventricles complete their depolarization, the wave returns to the iso-electric line. The downward deflection following the R wave is called the S wave when it goes below the iso-electric line. The QRS complex is the wave of ventricular depolarization.

A short iso-electric line follows—the ST segment—which represents early ventricular repolarization.

While the ventricles are depolarizing, the atria are repolarizing. The Ta wave of atrial repolarization is hidden.

Ventricular repolarization occurs from the epicardial to the endo-

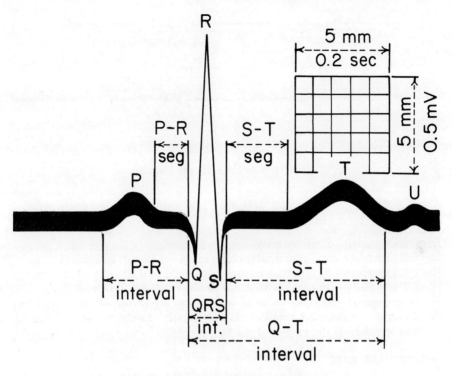

Fig. 8–7. Measuring complex components.

cardial surface. Taking this into account, along with the larger mass of the left ventricle, the resultant electrical force is again in the direction of the positive electrode. The T wave of ventricular repolarization is therefore upright in lead II. It is smaller and wider than the R wave, because repolarization is a slower process.

The U wave which follows the T wave is a low, round elevation. Authorities disagree as to the electrical cause of the U wave. Figures 8–5 and 8–6 show normal ECG patterns in bipolar, augmented and V leads.

The component waves and iso-electric portions of the whole cardiac cycle bear a mathematical relationship to each other, with established norms. An **interval** is a time measurement which includes a wave form. A **segment** is a time measurement which does not include a wave form.

See Figure 8–7 for normal interval and segment values. Bear in mind that as pulse rate increases, the shortening of the whole complex is chiefly in diastole, thereby shortening those measurements which pertain to repolarization.

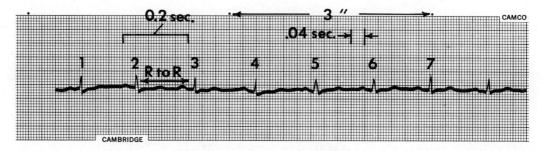

Fig. 8–8. How to calculate the heart rate.

Complexes, intervals and segments are measured from their convex curvatures. The normal ranges are:

1. P wave—atrial depolarization—up to 0.11 sec.
2. P-R interval—atrio-ventricular conduction—0.12 to 0.20 sec.
3. QRS complex—ventricular conduction—0.05 to 0.10 sec.
4. S-T segment—complete ventricular depolarization—0.14 to 0.16 sec.
5. Q-T interval—total duration of ventricular activation—0.33 to 0.43 sec.
6. T wave—ventricular repolarization—usually should be more than $\frac{1}{8}$ and less than $\frac{2}{3}$ the height of the R wave.

VENTRICULAR RATE

Figure 8–8 demonstrates how the heart rate may be calculated when the ventricular rate is regular—that is, if R-R intervals in the strip are equal in all cycles.

1. Measure the R-R interval in seconds and divide this figure into 60 seconds.
2. Count the number of small squares from R-R and divide into 1500 (1500 small squares equal 60 seconds).

If the ventricular rate is not regular—that is, if the P-R intervals in the strip are not equal in all cycles—do the following:

1. Count the number of R waves in a 6-inch strip and multiply by 10. Six inches of ECG strip represent 6 seconds.
2. Count the number of R waves in a 3-inch strip and multiply by 20. A 3-inch strip of ECG paper represents 3 seconds.

ATRIAL RATE

You may use the same methods as described above, using the P-P interval in place of the R-R interval.

REFERENCES AND BIBLIOGRAPHY

Bernreiter, M.: Electrocardiography. ed. 2. Philadelphia, J. B. Lippincott, 1963.

Burch, T., and Winsor, T.: A Primer of Electrocardiography. ed. 5. Philadelphia, Lea & Febiger, 1966.

Corday, E., and Irving, D. S.: Disturbances of Heart Rate, Rhythm, and Conduction. ed. 2. Philadelphia, W. B. Saunders, 1962.

Friedberg, C. K.: Diseases of the Heart. ed. 3. Philadelphia, W. B. Saunders, 1966.

Goldman, M. J.: Principles of Clinical Electrocardiography. ed. 6. Los Altos, California, Lange Medical Publications, 1967.

Guyton, A. C.: Textbook of Medical Physiology. ed. 3. Philadelphia, W. B. Saunders, 1968.

Jude, J. R., and Elam, J. O.: Fundamentals of Cardio-Pulmonary Resuscitation. Philadelphia, F. A. Davis, 1965.

Ritota, M.: Diagnostic Electrocardiography. Philadelphia, J. B. Lippincott, 1969.

Schaub, R.: Fundamentals of Clinical Electrocardiography. Switzerland, Documenta Geigy, 1966.

Wiggers, C. J.: The heart. Sci. Am., 62:11, 1960.

Wood, P.: Diseases of the Heart and Circulation. ed. 3. Philadelphia, J. B. Lippincott, 1968.

9 BASIC CONCEPTS OF ARRHYTHMIAS

Disturbances in the rate, rhythm and conduction of the heart's electrical impulses underlie the concept of arrhythmias. We shall now consider the chief concepts concerning physiological disturbances involving the arrhythmias.

PREMATURE BEATS

Premature beats are contractions of the whole or part of the heart muscle structure which occur earlier than expected in the patient's regular rhythm. The electrical impulse triggering the premature contraction arises in an area other than the S-A node. The area giving rise to the premature beat is called an *ectopic focus*. The ectopic focus triggers a premature contraction, actively or passively, when it finds heart muscle nonrefractory.

ACTIVE ECTOPIC FOCUS

Sometimes a cell or group of cells in the myocardium becomes more irritable than normal because its automatic rate has been increased by changes in the permeability of the cell membrane due to localized tissue damage, anoxia or the toxic effects of drugs. In this cell or group of cells, automaticity has been enhanced. If the ectopic focus rate of impulse formation is faster than that of the S-A node, it assumes the role of pacemaker for an isolated or occasional premature beat. If the ectopic focus retains its enhanced automaticity for longer periods, it assumes the role of pacemaker at its own rapid rate, as in the tachycardia of atrial and ventricular origins.

PASSIVE ECTOPIC FOCUS

The S-A node defaults when its impulse formation slows down or fails completely, or when there is failure to conduct the S-A nodal impulse to the atrial musculature because of block. By right of its now superior rate of automaticity, an ectopic focus takes over as pacemaker at its own intrinsic rate.

An **escape beat** is one which arises from another pacemaker impulse by default of the S-A node or other pacemaker. An **escape rhythm** is a series of escape beats.

Premature beats are classified according to site of origin:

1. **Supraventricular.** Those which arise from foci above the bifurcation of the bundle of His.
   a. *Sino-atrial.* Those which arise in the tail rather than in the head of the S-A node.
   b. *Atrial*
   c. *A-V junctional* (A-V nodal)
2. **Ventricular.** Those which arise from automatic foci anywhere in the left or right ventricle.

The depolarization wave from an ectopic focus goes radially from that focus. The ECG wave form differs from the normal to the extent the ectopic focus is distant from the normal S-A nodal site, and to the extent the muscle above the ectopic focus is stimulated by retrograde (backward) conduction from the ectopic site.

Premature beats can occur as isolated phenomena, with varying degrees of frequency, or may establish a mathematical relationship with the normal beat.

1. **Bigeminy,** or coupling—one normal to one abnormal
2. **Trigeminy**—one normal to two abnormal or two normal to one abnormal
3. **Quadrigeminy**—one normal to three abnormal or three normal to one abnormal

A **salvo** is five or more abnormal beats in succession. When several premature beats arise from the same focus, they are called *monotopic* or *unifocal.* When premature beats arise from more than one ectopic focus, they are called *polytopic* or *multifocal.*

When a normal rhythm is slow enough so that a premature beat does not wipe out the expected normal beat, we actually have one additional **interpolated** beat within a normal rhythm. The interpolated beat is the only true **extrasystole.**

Regardless of the location of the ectopic focus, the underlying mechanism is the same. Altered electrical pathways stimulate muscular contractions at variance in time and order from the normal, if the electrical impulse reaches muscle in its nonrefractory period.

Etiology

The cause of premature beats is not clearly defined. Premature beats have been recorded for which no cause could be discovered. Factors which seem to cause premature beats in some hearts do not do so in others. In all probability, combinations of factors are the trigger. Following is a list of such factors:

1. Direct stimulation to a surgically exposed heart
2. Abnormal process of impulse formation
3. Stimulation from hypothalamus
4. Organic heart disease
5. Reflex from abdominal organs
6. Infection
7. Hyperthyroidism
8. Drugs—digitalis, epinephrine, chloroform, ephedrine cyclopropane, barium chloride, tranquilizers
9. Common stimulants—coffee, tea, alcohol, tobacco
10. Emotional stress
11. Fatigue
12. Electrolyte imbalance
13. Cerebral tumors
14. Cardiac catheterization and angiography
15. Arteriosclerotic heart disease
16. Myocardial damage following infectious disease
17. Fluctuations of pH

The symptoms, significance, hemodynamic value and treatment will be discussed in chapters 10 and 11.

CONDUCTION BLOCK

The A-V node, common bundle, right and left bundle branches and Purkinje fibers are conductive pathways. Actual tissue death, anoxia, fibrosis or control from the central nervous system can slow or stop passage of electrical impulse along these pathways.

MECHANISMS IN CONDUCTION BLOCK

1. **Physiological.** In rapid atrial tachycardia at rates over 200, the refractory period of the conducting tissue at the A-V junction will not shorten sufficiently to allow passage of each impulse.
2. **Interference**
   a. If two pacemakers in different areas of the heart discharge almost simultaneously, their excitation waves travel toward each other. Each wave encounters tissue which has been made refractory by the other wave, and one impulse cancels out the other. This is interference block.
   b. Following a ventricular extrasystole with retrograde conduction through the A-V node, the following sinus impulse may be blocked from being conducted through to the ventricles by refractoriness of the A-V node. This is interference block.

3. **Aberrant conduction.** A rapid supraventricular pacemaker impulse may find one of the bundle branches refractory. Intraventricular conduction will be disturbed, and the QRS presents a pattern resembling bundle branch block. This is aberrant conduction.

4. **Entrance block.** An ectopic pacemaker at a slower rate than the S-A node discharges independently and activates nonrefractory myocardium. Some mechanism, not clearly understood, protects the ectopic impulse from being inhibited by the faster pacemaker. This type of ectopic beat is called *parasystole*. Two rhythms are operating in parallel. To qualify as parasystole, there must be:
   a. Wide variations in coupling time with preceding beats
   b. The time intervals between ectopic beats must bear a mathematical relationship to each other, usually being exact multiples of the ectopic pacemaker rate.
   c. From time to time, the dominant pacemaker and the ectopic pacemaker rhythm impulses must invade the same myocardial area, and the result of the two impulses gives rise to a *fusion beat*. The contour of the fusion beat must be intermediate between the contour of the dominant beat and the ectopic beat.

5. **Exit block.** An ectopic pacemaker at a slower rate than the S-A node discharges independently, but impulses do not always invade the surrounding myocardium, even when the surrounding myocardium could be expected to be nonrefractory. The exact mechanism for this block is not clear. One explanation is that the ectopic discharging rate is actually higher than appears in the ECG, and that the rapid discharging rate keeps the surrounding tissue refractory so that the ectopic impulse is not conducted.

6. **Re-entry.** The A-V junction is normally capable of conducting a stimulus in either direction, but occasionally unidirectional block occurs. On rare occasions, unidirectional block occurs in only a portion of the A-V junction, and the remainder is capable of conduction in both directions.

   In a junctional rhythm, a junctional impulse which has activated the atria by retrograde conduction may re-enter part of the junction and be conducted back to the ventricle, thereby producing a second ventricular contraction. This is called a *reciprocal beat*.

7. **Concealed, or decremental, conduction.** If a stimulus reaches any part of conducting tissue before repolarization is complete, the transmembrane potential is low. If the transmembrane potential has reached two thirds of normal resting level, conduction can occur but will be slower than normal. As this impulse passes along conduction pathways, it becomes blocked. While this weak action current produces no change in the ECG, it leaves refractory tissue in its wake. This concealed conduction affects the transmission of the next impulse since it encounters refractory tissue.

CLASSIFICATION OF CARDIAC ARRHYTHMIAS

The integrity of the normal electrical cardiac cycle depends upon:

1. Normal impulse formation (pacemaking)
2. Normal pathways of excitation (conduction)

Table 9–1 lists the arrhythmias which will be discussed in detail in the following two chapters.

TABLE 9–1. CLASSIFICATION OF CARDIAC ARRHYTHMIAS

SITE OF DISORDER	DISORDER OF IMPULSE FORMATION	DISORDER OF IMPULSE CONDUCTION
S-A node	Sinus bradycardia Sinus tachycardia Sinus arrest Atrial standstill	S-A block
Atria	Premature atrial contractions Atrial tachycardia Atrial flutter Atrial fibrillation Wandering pacemaker	Intra-atrial block

A-V node	Premature nodal
	   contractions
	Nodal rhythm
	Nodal tachycardia
		A-V dissociation
		
		Interference dissociation
		Fusion beats
		A-V blocks
		   1st degree
		   2nd degree
		      Wenckebach
		         (Mobitz 1)
		      Mobitz 2
		   3rd degree

Bundle branch		Bundle branch block
		   left—complete
		      and partial
		   right—complete
		      and partial
		   bilateral

Ventricles	Premature ventricular contractions Ventricular tachycardia Ventricular fibrillation Idio-ventricular rhythm Ventricular standstill	
Purkinje network		Arborization block

DETECTING ARRHYTHMIAS IN AN ECG STRIP

The nurse should proceed in a logical sequence to determine the presence or absence of arrhythmia in an ECG strip.

An arrhythmia manifests itself in altered contours or absence of waves, in altered timing, altered positivity or negativity and altered precedence of wave forms. The use of calipers is a quick method of comparing time intervals and voltages of wave forms from cycle to cycle.

The Lansing ECG rule (devised by Dr. Peter R. Lansing) is a transparent ruler, the sides of which are calibrated in normal ranges of P-R, QRS and Q-T intervals. One border is inscribed with a scale for rapid calculation of the heart rate. Some pharmaceutical houses give modifications of this useful instrument as part of their advertising campaign.

Following is a suggested sequence for examination of a strip of lead II:

1. **Basic rhythm**
   The patient's basic rhythm need not be normal. Compare your strip with previous recordings. An atrial ectopic beat with a bundle branch block may look like a premature ventricular beat, because the QRS is wide.
2. **P waves**
   Are they present, before or after QRS, positive or negative in deflection, normal in contour, up to 0.10 sec. in duration?
   If a positive P wave, normal in contour, is present before each QRS, the rhythm is normal sinus.
   In lead II, if P waves are absent, negative in deflection, abnormal in contour, or following the QRS, an ectopic pacemaker is operative.
   If the P waves are absent, does the base line undulate or have sawtooth configuration? If so, then atrial flutter or fibrillation is present.
3. **QRS**
   If the QRS is absent following a P wave, A-V block may be present. Remember that a QRS can precede the P wave in an ectopic pacemaker.
   If the QRS is 0.12 sec. or longer in duration, conduction in the ventricles is disturbed.
   If the QRS falls too soon, is wide, slurred, notched or bizarre in appearance and does not follow a P wave, this is a premature ventricular beat.
   A sudden pronounced prolongation of QRS signifies the patient's life is in danger.
4. **P-P interval**
   If the P-P interval is irregular, there is a possibility of sinus arrhythmia or wandering pacemaker.
   If the P-P interval prolongs to approximate multiples of the P-P interval of the basic rhythm, sinus arrest or S-A block may be present.

If the P wave falls too soon in the basic rhythm, this indicates a probable premature atrial beat.

5. **R-R interval**

What is the ventricular rate? If less than 60, bradycardia is indicated; if more than 100, tachycardia is indicated.

If the atrial rate is greater than the ventricular rate, this indicates that all atrial stimuli are not being conducted to the ventricles.

If the R wave falls too soon, this indicates a premature beat.

6. **P-R interval**

Normal is 0.12 to 0.20 sec. If prolonged, atrio-ventricular conduction is disturbed. If reduced, is it a normal sinus beat?

Is the patient on digitalis or antiarrhythmic drugs?

If P-R interval progressively prolongs beat-to-beat, watch for a Wenckebach type of A-V block.

Some arrhythmias cannot be definitely diagnosed in lead II. Where P waves seem to be absent in lead II, they may be evident in other leads. Look at the full ECG. Discuss it with the patient's physician. Never be reluctant to ask for advice or information.

REFERENCES AND BIBLIOGRAPHY

Bernreiter, M.: Electrocardiography. ed. 2. Philadelphia, J. B. Lippincott, 1963.

Burch, T., and Winsor, T.: A Primer of Electrocardiography. ed. 5. Philadelphia, Lea & Febiger, 1966.

Corday, E., and Irving, D. S.: Disturbances of Heart Rate, Rhythm, and Conduction. ed. 2. Philadelphia, W. B. Saunders, 1962.

Friedberg, C. K.: Diseases of the Heart. ed. 3. Philadelphia, W. B. Saunders, 1966.

Goldman, M. J.: Principles of Clinical Electrocardiography. ed. 6. Los Altos, California, Lange Medical Publications, 1967.

Guyton, A. C.: Textbook of Medical Physiology. ed. 3. Philadelphia, W. B. Saunders, 1968.

Jude, J. R., Elam, J. O.: Fundamentals of Cardio-Pulmonary Resuscitation. Philadelphia, F. A. Davis, 1965.

Ritota, M.: Diagnostic Electrocardiography. Philadelphia, J. B. Lippincott, 1969.

Schaub, R.: Fundamentals of Clinical Electrocardiography. Switzerland, Documenta Geigy, 1966.

Stock, J. P. P.: Diagnosis and Treatment of Cardiac Arrhythmias. New York, Appleton-Century-Crofts, 1969.

Wiggers, C. J.: The Heart. Sci. Am. 62:11. 1960.

Wood, P.: Diseases of the Heart and Circulation. ed. 3. Philadelphia, J. B. Lippincott, 1968.

10 CARDIAC ARRHYTHMIAS: DISORDERS OF IMPULSE FORMATION

Normally the electrical impulse is initiated in the S-A node. This chapter discusses those disorders resulting from disturbances in impulse formation. The material is presented according to the sites at which these disorders originate, namely the S-A node, the atrium, the A-V node and the ventricles.

SINO-ATRIAL NODE

The disorders in impulse formation arising in the S-A node are sinus bradycardia, sinus tachycardia, sinus arrest, and atrial standstill.

Sinus Arrhythmia

Sinus arrhythmia is a common variation of normal sinus rhythm in which the rate alternately increases and decreases due to alternations of vagal tone, with direct effect on S-A node impulse formation. The variations are usually related to the respiratory cycle, the rate increasing with inspiration and decreasing with expiration.

ETIOLOGY
1. Exaggeration of the normal rate control mechanism of the heart
2. Though benign, sinus arrhythmia is sometimes present in fevers, infectious diseases, valvular and coronary heart disease and disease states which produce increased intracranial pressure.

CLINICAL ASPECTS
1. Sinus arrhythmia produces no symptoms or hemodynamic upset.
2. It is most common at slow heart rates, when vagal forces are maximal.
3. The arrhythmia can be intensified by deep inspiration and abolished by holding the breath.

111

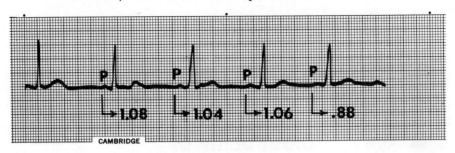

FIG. 10–1. Sinus arrhythmia.

ECG FINDINGS

1. P waves are normal.
2. Each P wave is followed by a normal QRS.
3. The longest and shortest P-P interval must differ by at least 0.12 second.

TREATMENT

None

NURSING RESPONSIBILITIES

Identify and document, by ECG strip, as sinus arrhythmia.

Figure 10–1 is an example of sinus arrhythmia. Each P wave is followed by a normal QRS. The P-P interval in this strip is changing constantly. The difference between the fastest and slowest P-P is 0.2 second.

Sinus Bradycardia

Sinus bradycardia is characterized by a regular pulse rate of 60 or less. The S-A node is the pacemaker. Conduction is normal, as is ventricular response. The slow rate is ascribed to increased vagal tone, decreased sympathetic tone, or a combination of both. Increased susceptibility of ischemic myocardium to vagotonia can be a contributing factor.

ETIOLOGY

1. Athlete's heart
2. Factors increasing vagal tone, such as increased intracranial pressure, increased intraabdominal pressure or carotid sinus stimulation
3. Factors increasing sympathetic tone
4. Hypothyroidism
5. Toxins—mushroom poisoning, infectious diseases
6. Myocardial infarction
7. Drugs—digitalis, narcotics, reserpine, anesthetic agents

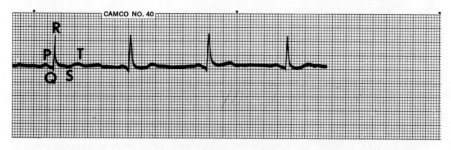

FIG. 10-2. Sinus bradycardia.

HEMODYNAMICS

Normal or high systolic blood pressure with low diastolic (wide pulse-pressure)

CLINICAL ASPECTS

1. There may be no signs or symptoms other than slow rate.
2. In very slow rates, there may be palpitation, dyspnea, dizziness, chest pain or syncope.
3. Bradycardia under anesthesia may be a precursor of serious arrhythmia or even cardiac arrest.
4. In myocardial infarction, very slow bradycardia may be a precursor of A-V block or of serious ventricular arrhythmia.

ECG FINDINGS

1. P waves are normal in configuration and fall regularly.
2. P-P interval is 1.0 second or more.
3. Each P wave is followed by a normal QRS.
4. A full ECG must be done to exclude diagnosis of slow nodal rhythm or heart block.

TREATMENT

1. Usually none
2. Atropine to decrease vagal tone
3. Discontinue incriminated drugs.
4. Accelerator stimulation by ephedrine-like drugs if slow rate cannot be tolerated

NURSING RESPONSIBILITIES

1. Identify and document with an ECG.
2. Check vital signs.
3. Check apical and radial rate for pulse deficit.
4. Assess clinical state.

5. Chart findings.
6. Notify physician if symptoms develop or if another pacemaker takes over.

Figure 10–2 is an example of sinus bradycardia. P waves are normal and regular, and each is followed by a QRS. The atrial and ventricular rates are identical at 52. The P-P interval is 1.12 seconds.

Sinus Tachycardia

Sinus tachycardia is a disturbance of heart rate, characterized by a pulse rate over 100, due to decreased vagal tone, increased sympathetic tone, or a combination of both. There is a normal sinus node pacemaker and conduction. The ventricular responses are normal.

ETIOLOGY

1. Physiological response to pain, emotional stress, exercise or gastric dilatation
2. Response to body need for more cardiac output, as in shock, hemorrhage, anemia or cardiac failure
3. Febrile or infectious diseases
4. Hyperthyroidism, pheochromocytoma
5. Drugs—atropine, ephedrine, amphetamine
6. Common stimulants such as tea, coffee, tobacco or alcohol

HEMODYNAMICS

1. Normal or increased cardiac output and coronary blood flow at rates up to 180 in normal hearts
2. In partial or complete coronary occlusion, the coronary flow cannot increase to provide adequate perfusion of the myocardium.

CLINICAL ASPECTS

1. The patient may or may not complain of palpitation, dyspnea or fatigue.
2. Apical and radial pulses are identical at a rate above 100, though rarely exceeding 160.
3. Sinus tachycardia is gradual in onset and termination.
4. Chest pain may occur at rapid rates.
5. Must be distinguished from atrial tachycardia by an ECG. This distinction is sometimes difficult to make.
6. If coronary disease is present, signs of congestive heart failure may develop.

ECG FINDINGS

1. P waves are normal in configuration, upright in lead II and fall regularly at a rate above 100.

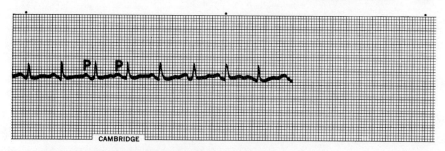

Fig. 10–3. Sinus tachycardia.

2. P-P interval is less than 0.6 second.
3. QRS is of normal configuration after each P wave.
4. The time reduction in the individual cardiac cycle is chiefly in diastole. In rates over 150, the P wave may fuse with the preceding T wave.

TREATMENT
1. Sedation
2. Withdrawal of incriminated drugs or stimulants
3. Treatment of underlying condition

NURSING RESPONSIBILITIES
1. Identify and document with an ECG.
2. Record time of onset.
3. Check vital signs—blood pressure, apical pulse, radial pulse, respirations.
4. Assess clinical condition—pain, pallor, diaphoresis, cyanosis, emotional state.
5. Give sedation if indicated and if ordered by the physician.
6. Notify physician.

Figure 10–3 shows the monitor strip of a 58-year-old woman who was admitted to the emergency room with complaints of weakness, dizziness, faintness and chest pain of several hours duration. Blood pressure was 110/80, pulse rate, 110 to 120, and temperature, normal. The only ECG changes were those of sinus tachycardia—normal P-QRS at a regular rate of 120.

The patient was given Demerol, 75 mg., for pain, admitted to the coronary care unit, and monitored. Very apprehensive on admission, the patient became much calmer when her pain was relieved. Subsequent ECG's proved an acute anterior myocardial infarction. She developed no rhythm problems or signs of failure, and went on to uncomplicated convalescence.

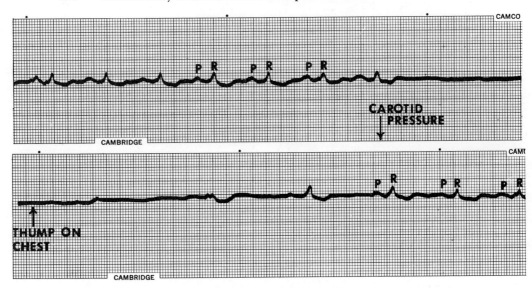

Fig. 10–4. Induced sinus arrest.

Sinus Arrest

Sinus arrest is a disturbance of pacemaker function in which vagal suppression or disease of the S-A node causes failure of the node to initiate an electrical impulse. There is no stimulation to atria or ventricles, and therefore no P, QRS, T or muscle response. The duration of the pause is not a multiple of the normal cycle length. In short pauses, the S-A node usually resumes the role of pacemaker with the succeeding beat. Where the pause is long, an escape pacemaker in the junctional area or in the ventricles will take over. It may be impossible to distinguish sinus arrest from S-A block, which will be discussed later.

ETIOLOGY
1. Increased vagal tone
2. Digitalis toxicity
3. Quinidine toxicity
4. S-A node disease—infarction

CLINICAL ASPECTS
1. In short pauses, the patient may or may not be aware of the dropped beat.
2. In longer pauses, the patient may complain of dizziness or faintness.
3. In still longer pauses, all the symptoms and findings of cardiac arrest will be evident.

ECG FINDINGS

1. There is a pause between the PQRS's though the length of the pause is not an exact multiple of the normal distance between cycles.
2. Following short pauses, there is a resumption of normal sinus rhythm.
3. Longer pauses may terminate in nodal escape (inverted P wave before or after normal QRS, or a normal QRS with an absent P wave).
4. Still longer pauses may terminate in ventricular escape (an absent P wave with an abnormal QRS).

TREATMENT

1. In short pauses, none
2. Atropine to reduce vagal tone
3. Isoproterenol
4. Ephedrine to stimulate sympathetic tone
5. Treatment of cardiac arrest in prolonged asystole

NURSING RESPONSIBILITIES

1. Identify and document with an ECG.
2. Notify physician if episodes increase in number or duration.
3. Withhold digitalis, quinidine or sedatives pending physician's advice.
4. Be prepared for pacemaking or resuscitation.

Figure 10–4 demonstrates induced sinus arrest. In a run of normal sinus rhythm, prolonged asystole is induced by carotid pressure. The asystole was terminated by a sharp blow to the chest (Fig. 10–4, *bottom*). Ventricular and nodal beats precede the resumption of normal sinus rhythm.

Atrial Standstill

Atrial standstill is the absence of atrial activity for one or more beats, but with the ventricles continuing to contract regularly in response to secondary or tertiary pacemakers.

Due to failure of the S-A node to initiate an electrical impulse (sinus arrest), or failure of the S-A node to conduct an electrical impulse to the atria (S-A block), there is no electrical or muscular activity in the atria.

The standstill may terminate by one of the following means:

1. A-V nodal escape beat, with resumption of normal sinus rhythm
2. A-V nodal escape rhythm, with no retrograde conduction to atria
3. Ventricular escape beat, with resumption of normal sinus rhythm
4. Ventricular escape rhythm
5. Cardiac arrest

Note: The same factors which have disabled the primary pacemaker may progressively involve the secondary and tertiary pacemakers, leaving the heart with no pacemaker to sustain life.

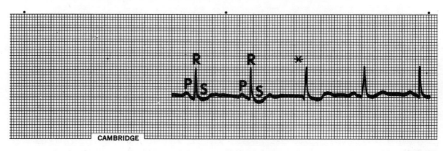

FIG. 10–5. Atrial standstill.

ETIOLOGY

1. Organic heart disease
2. Coronary heart disease
3. Vagal stimulation
4. Hyperkalemia

HEMODYNAMICS

If normal sinus rhythm is resumed very quickly, there is little or no hemodynamic upset. If another pacemaker takes over, the hemodynamic values are those of the capturing rhythm.

CLINICAL ASPECTS

Momentary standstill of the atria produces no typical signs or symptoms. Diagnosis is made by an ECG. If either the A-V node or the ventricle takes over as pacemaker, the symptoms are those of the secondary or tertiary pacemaker rhythm. If no other pacemaker takes over, the symptoms are those of cardiac arrest.

If the arrhythmia is due to drug toxicity or hyperkalemia, it is potentially reversible. If it is due to severe myocardial damage, the prognosis is grave.

ECG FINDINGS

1. Absence of P waves
2. QRS regular, except in the dying heart
   a. Normal in contour if A-V node is the pacemaker
   b. Wide and bizarre if ventricular pacemaker

TREATMENT

1. Discontinue suspect drugs.
2. Correct hyperkalemia by:
   a. I.V. glucose with insulin
   b. Restricting potassium intake

c. Ion exchange resins
d. Dialysis
3. Use artificial pacemaking.
4. Perform resuscitative procedure if cardiac arrest.

NURSING RESPONSIBILITIES
1. Identify and document with an ECG.
2. Notify physician.
3. Turn on stand-by pacemaker if adequate pacemaker does not take over.

Figure 10–5 shows atrial standstill. The third QRS in this strip is not associated with a P wave. The QRS itself is normal. Except for the dropped P wave, the P-P intervals undergo no change. This is most likely nonconduction with no contraction in the atria. Conduction is probably through specialized atrial tracts to the A-V node. This strip demonstrates atrial standstill for the duration of one beat.

ATRIAL ECTOPIC PACEMAKER
The disorders in impulse formation arising in the atria are premature atrial beats, atrial tachycardia, atrial flutter, atrial fibrillation and wandering pacemaker.

Premature Atrial Beat (PAB)
A premature atrial beat is a disturbance of impulse formation, characterized by a beat which comes earlier than expected in the basic rhythm.

An irritable ectopic focus in the atrium initiates an early beat. This premature atrial beat depolarizes the S-A node by retrograde conduction, and the S-A node becomes refractory. This delays the next normal sinus impulse. The premature atrial beat is then followed by a pause before the next normal beat. The elapsed time of one normal beat plus the succeeding premature beat is less than the elapsed time of two normal successive beats. The pause following the premature atrial beat is not fully compensated.

If the premature impulse reaches the A-V node at its refractory period, it may not be conducted to the ventricle, or the ventricular muscle may still be refractory, and thus no ventricular response will occur. There will be a dropped beat—a blocked premature atrial beat.

ETIOLOGY
Factors which prolong the nonrefractory period (called the vulnerable period) tend to allow premature atrial beats to occur. The incidence of premature atrial beats is higher in heart disease with atrial enlargement, such as mitral stenosis or cor pulmonale.

Such beats occur often in healthy hearts as well as in all kinds of organic heart disease. They may result from emotional stress or from the use of common stimulants.

HEMODYNAMICS

When the premature atrial beat occurs sufficiently early so that the ventricles have not had a chance to fill, the resulting contraction may be diminished in force or stroke volume. Isolated PAB's cause little, if any, hemodynamic upset.

CLINICAL ASPECTS

The patient may or may not be aware of the premature beat. The difference in pulse force may be perceptible at the wrist. The absence of ventricular response to the blocked PAB may be noted at the wrist or at the apex.

ECG FINDINGS

1. The P wave occurs early in the basic rhythm.
2. In lead II, if the ectopic focus is high in the atrium, the P wave is positive in deflection. If low in the atrium, near the A-V node, the P wave is negative in deflection.
3. Each P wave is followed by a QRS, except in the blocked premature atrial beat.
4. The QRS complex is that of the basic rhythm. That is to say, if ventricular conduction is normal in the basic rhythm, it will be normal in the PAB, unless there is aberrant conduction.
5. The R-R interval of the normal beat added to the R-R interval of the PAB does not equal two normal R-R intervals.
6. The T wave of the preceding beat may be distorted by the P wave of the premature beat, if it falls early enough.

TREATMENT

1. Elimination of stress
2. Adequate rest
3. Sedation, if necessary
4. Treatment of underlying disease
5. Elimination of incriminated drugs or stimulants
6. Antiarrhythmic drugs if more than six PAB's per minute

NURSING RESPONSIBILITIES

1. Identify and document with an ECG.
2. Check clinical condition and vital signs.
3. Reassure patient.

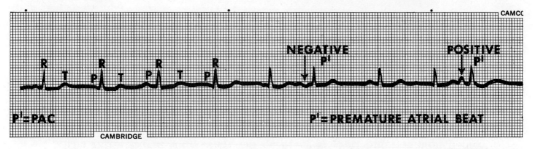

FIG. 10–6. Premature atrial beat.

4. Chart findings.
5. Notify the physician if incidence increases or if there are more than six PAB's per minute. Such contractions may herald atrial tachycardia, fibrillation or flutter, particularly with underlying heart disease.

Figure 10–6 presents premature atrial beats. The sixth R wave falls early and is preceded by a negative P wave. The ninth R wave falls early and is preceded by a positive P wave. The QRS is normal. The P-R interval is greater than 0.10 second. The R-R interval from beat 7 to beat 8 is 19 small squares. The R-R from beat 8 to beat 10 is 37 small squares, i.e., one small square less than the sum of two normal R-R intervals.

Paroxysmal Atrial Tachycardia (PAT)

Paroxysmal atrial tachycardia is a disturbance of impulse formation characterized by a rapid, regular rate of 140–220. An irritable focus in the atrium, other than the S-A node, triggers a sudden burst of six or more premature atrial beats, with normal ventricular response. It may be heralded and followed by occasional premature atrial beats of the same configuration as the rapid beats. The rate slows as suddenly as it speeds up. The rapid rate may vary in duration from seconds to hours or even days.

ETIOLOGY

1. May occur in healthy hearts
2. Emotional stress
3. Mitral valve disease
4. Hyperthyroidism
5. Coronary heart disease
6. Incidental to cardiac catheterization or surgery
7. Drugs—thyroid, diuretics, digitalis
8. Common stimulants—caffeine, alcohol, tobacco
9. Wolf-Parkinson-White syndrome

HEMODYNAMICS

As the cardiac rate goes above 180 in normal hearts (less in diseased hearts), there is poor ventricular filling, resulting in decreased cardiac output. Central venous pressure rises and hypotension follows. This circulatory failure results in poor perfusion of all vital organs.

The degree of hemodynamic upset depends upon the underlying heart condition. Cardiac failure can be induced even in healthy hearts if the atrial tachycardia continues for days. The average reduction of coronary blood flow at rapid rates is 35 to 60 per cent. This makes atrial tachycardia a dangerous rhythm in coronary heart disease.

CLINICAL ASPECTS

There may be no symptoms, or the patient may complain of palpitation, chest pain, dyspnea, dizziness or faintness. The radial pulse is rapid and regular, unless A-V block develops. The neck veins may be distended and pulsating with the heartbeat if cardiac failure sets in. Bowel distention often accompanies the attack. If there is underlying heart disease, congestive heart failure may develop rapidly. The patient may progress to shock with hypotension, cyanosis and cold clammy skin.

ECG FINDINGS

1. P waves are present at a regular rate of 140–220. If the ectopic focus is high in the atrium, the P waves are positive in deflection; if low in the atrium, negative in deflection. The contour of the P wave may differ from the P wave of normal sinus rhythm.
2. A normal QRS follows each P wave, unless there is disturbed intraventricular conduction.
3. In very rapid rates, P waves may fuse with the preceding T wave.
4. The S-T depression and T wave inversion of ischemia may appear during the attack and last for several days.
5. Occasionally, ischemia or fatigue of atrio-ventricular conduction results in block in which not all beats are conducted to the ventricles. A QRS may follow every second, third or fourth P wave, or the response may become completely irregular.

TREATMENT

1. **Preventive:**
   a. Treatment of thyrotoxicosis
   b. Avoidance of tea, coffee, tobacco and alcohol
   c. Sedation
   d. Digitalis, quinidine, propranolol, procainamide

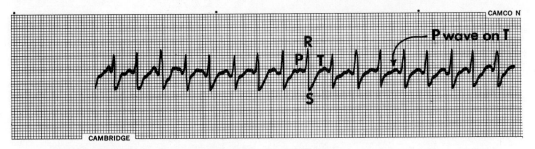

FIG. 10–7. Atrial tachycardia.

2. **Acute attack:**
   a. Sedation
   b. Reasurrance
   c. Oxygen
   d. Physician may attempt to increase vagal tone by eyeball pressure, gagging, Valsalva's maneuver or carotid sinus massage. Patients subject to PAT often discover that they can abort an attack by inducing vomiting. Carotid sinus massage can result in dangerous cerebral ischemia or in cardiac arrest, especially in the elderly patient.
   e. Digitalis increases vagal tone, slows A-V conduction and ventricular rate.
   f. Quinidine slows atrial rate and increases the refractory period.
   g. Vasopressors. Systolic pressure should not be allowed to rise above 180; otherwise other arrhythmias may be introduced, or a cerebrovascular accident may occur.

NURSING RESPONSIBILITIES

1. Identify and document with an ECG. Paroxysmal atrial tachycardia has a sudden onset and sudden termination, whereas sinus tachycardia has a gradual onset and gradual termination. Find the P wave to differentiate between PAT and ventricular tachycardia. If necessary, run a full ECG.
2. Record time of onset.
3. Assess clinical condition and check vital signs.
4. Notify physician immediately.
5. Give medication as ordered.
6. Be prepared to countershock.

Figure 10–7 presents atrial tachycardia. The P waves are slightly abnormal, followed by a normal QRS. The P-R interval is short. The R-R interval is regular at a rate of 170. The P waves often fuse with the T wave of the preceding complex.

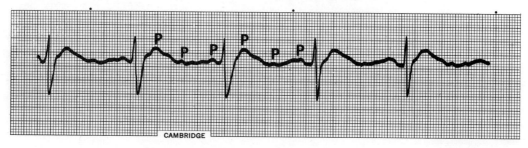

FIG. 10–8. Atrial tachycardia with 3:1 block.

Figure 10–8 is an example of atrial tachycardia with 3:1 block. There are three P waves between each QRS. The P waves differ slightly from each other. The first P wave following the QRS is somewhat fused with the preceding T wave. The QRS is prolonged to 0.12 second. The atrial rate is 138. The ventricular rate is 46.

This rhythm strip was taken on a 65-year-old man who was admitted to a medical unit with chest pain, dyspnea and signs of early congestive failure. He was placed on digitalis. Twenty-four hours later he suddenly developed a rapid heart rate and was transferred to the coronary care unit for monitoring. Subsequent ECG's showed a posterior myocardial infarction.

The patient showed increasing signs of congestive failure, and digitalis was continued. Blood pressure fell markedly and had to be maintained with Levophed. The patient then began to throw many premature ventricular beats, followed by a slow bigeminy. Digitalis was discontinued as a probable causative factor, and lidocaine by I.V. drip was started. The patient then went into complete heart block, with a very slow ventricular rate. A transvenous bipolar electrode catheter was passed and attached to a demand pacemaker. The patient returned to normal sinus rhythm in five days, and the catheter pacemaker was removed. He was transferred out of the CCU the following day, and went on to uncomplicated convalescence.

Atrial Flutter

Atrial flutter is a disturbance of pacemaker function characterized by a rapid, regular atrial rate of 250–350 (usually around 300), with varying degrees of block at the A-V node, so that the ventricles respond to every second, third, fourth or fifth atrial stimulus. In some cases, the response is completely irregular.

In atrial flutter in the exposed heart, the rapid vibrations of the atria resemble the motion of a bird's wings in flight—hence the name "flutter."

Atrial flutter usually begins with a premature atrial beat. When the ectopic focus discharges faster than the S-A node, it assumes the role of pacemaker. As it speeds up further, the A-V node becomes blocked due to refractoriness. The "saw-tooth" pattern of atrial flutter arises as follows:

The Ta wave of atrial repolarization is not usually seen in lead II because it is hidden in the larger electrical complexes. As the ectopic atrial rate increases, the Ta wave becomes visible and is followed by an iso-electric line. As the rate increases further, the iso-electric line becomes shorter and shorter. The saw-tooth pattern consists of a P wave, a discordant Ta wave and a very, very short iso-electric line.

ETIOLOGY

Atrial flutter is a much less common arrhythmia than atrial fibrillation. It occurs most often in older patients and in the presence of organic heart disease. It is associated with the following:

1. Rheumatic heart disease—mitral stenosis
2. Congenital heart disease
3. Coronary and hypertensive heart disease
4. Hyperthyroidism
5. Digitalis or quinidine toxicity
6. Myocardial infarction
7. Cardiac surgery
8. Febrile and infectious diseases
9. Conditions in which the atria become overdistended

HEMODYNAMICS

If a high degree of block exists, and the ventricular response to the rapid flutter is slow, there is little dynamic upset. If the ventricular response is a rapid one, the hemodynamic effects are the same as those of paroxysmal atrial tachycardia.

CLINICAL ASPECTS

The diagnosis must be made by ECG. It is paroxysmal in about one fifth of the cases. If it lasts longer than two weeks, it is spoken of as "established atrial flutter."

The symptoms become more acute as the rate of ventricular response becomes more rapid. There may be palpitation, nausea, weakness, dizziness, dyspnea, syncope, irregular radial pulse with pulse deficit, fear of impending death, anginal pain, hypotension and signs of congestive heart failure.

Acute pulmonary edema may appear at the onset of atrial flutter. Either atrial fibrillation or embolization may develop. Atrial flutter with a rapid ventricular rate in the presence of coronary heart disease is an emergency.

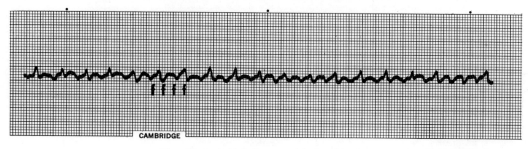

Fig. 10–9. Atrial flutter with 2:1 block.

ECG FINDINGS

1. Saw-tooth pattern
2. F waves of uniform size and shape, and regular in frequency
3. Absence of iso-electric line
4. R-R interval is usually constant, but can vary in varying block.
5. In rapid atrial flutter with 1:2 or 2:1 conduction, the pattern may resemble a series of QRS complexes in ventricular tachycardia.

TREATMENT

1. Cardioversion
2. Digitalis to slow ventricular rate and prevent failure. Note that digitalis may convert atrial flutter to atrial fibrillation.
3. Quinidine, when heart rate has been slowed
4. Procainamide—rarely
5. Sedation
6. Avoidance of stimulants

NURSING RESPONSIBILITIES

1. Identify and document with an ECG.
2. Notify physician.
3. Assess clinical condition and check vital signs.
4. Give medication as ordered. If digitalis is given, be alert for digitalis-induced atrial fibrillation.
5. Be prepared to assist with cardioversion.

Figure 10–9 presents atrial flutter with 2:1 block. Flutter waves are present at a rate of 340. There is no iso-electric line. The QRS is regular at a rate of 170. Only every other atrial impulse is being conducted to the ventricles. The saw-tooth characteristics of this arrhythmia would be more evident if this strip had been run on double standardization. Doubling the voltage would have increased the amplitude of the whole complex and would have made the flutter waves more distinct.

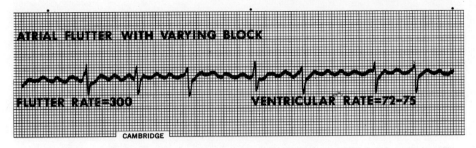

Fig. 10–10. Atrial flutter with varying block.

Figure 10–10 presents atrial flutter with varying block. Flutter waves are at a rate of 300. The number of flutter waves between QRS varies from two to five. The ventricular response is irregular at a rate of 72–75. Note the saw-tooth configuration.

Atrial Fibrillation

After premature ventricular contraction, atrial fibrillation is the most common arrhythmia. It is a disturbance of impulse formation characterized by a very rapid atrial rate. It has a close affinity to atrial flutter. It is not uncommon to see combinations or alternations of these arrhythmias in the same patient. It can be chronic or paroxysmal, lasting from several hours to several days.

The impulse for atrial fibrillation arises in irritable ectopic foci in the atria. This gives rise to very rapid, chaotic atrial activity (350–600/min.), with irregular conduction to the ventricles.

ETIOLOGY
1. Arteriosclerotic heart disease and myocardial infarction
2. Hypertensive heart disease
3. Hyperthyroidism
4. Chronic pericarditis
5. Pulmonary embolization
6. Heart failure
7. Atrial-septal defects
8. Mitral disease
9. Incidental to A-V block
10. Incidental to cardiac catheterization and angiography
11. Incidental to open-heart surgery

HEMODYNAMICS
Hemodynamic effects are related to the rate of ventricular response and the duration of the arrhythmia. There is some decrease in cardiac output due to the loss of atrial transport.

At rapid ventricular rates, the ventricles are not able to fill properly, resulting in reduced output and poor perfusion of vital organs. Cerebral blood flow diminishes as much as 23 per cent, coronary blood flow as much as 40 per cent. Circulation time is prolonged, central venous pressure rises, and circulatory shock and cardiac failure may develop. Where cerebral and coronary artery circulation is already compromised by arteriosclerotic changes, the prognosis for atrial fibrillation is poor.

Thrombus formation in the dilated atria is common. Portions of this thrombus can break off and pass into the general circulation as emboli.

CLINICAL ASPECTS

There is a rapid, irregular atrial rate of 350–600 per minute. The ventricular rate may be over 100. Ventricular rates of less than 60 can be found in older patients or in those on digitalis therapy. There is a pulse deficit, and variations of pulse force can be felt at the wrist.

The symptoms increase in severity as the rate of ventricular response increases. At slow rates, there may be few if any symptoms. Many people with chronic atrial fibrillation with a slow ventricular response are able to live fairly active lives. When atrial fibrillation with a rapid ventricular response persists in the presence of underlying heart disease, it will probably lead to heart failure.

At the onset of paroxysmal atrial fibrillation, the patient may be pale and may complain of palpitation, nausea and weakness.

ECG FINDINGS

1. Polymorphic P waves and very frequent extrasystoles are usually forerunners of atrial fibrillation.
2. P waves are absent. Small, irregular waves (fibrillatory waves) appear and are characterized by continuously changing voltage, shape and frequency.
3. The QRS of the basic rhythm appears irregularly because some degree of A-V block is present.
4. The ventricular rate may be over 100 or less than 60. The ventricular response in chronic atrial fibrillation is much slower than that of the paroxysmal type, mainly because of treatment.

TREATMENT

The course of treatment is determined by the severity of symptoms and the degree to which circulation is compromised.
1. **Chronic atrial fibrillation:**
   a. Digitalis to slow A-V conduction and increase force of ventricular contraction
   b. Quinidine for premature ventricular contractions or to convert to normal sinus rhythm. It reduces myocardial irritability, prolongs refractory time and slows conduction. It should be discontinued if the QRS widens to more than 0.12 second or if complete heart

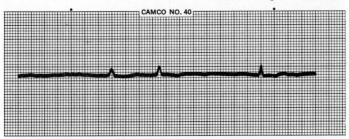

FIG. 10–11. Atrial fibrillation with slow ventricular response.

block develops. Ventricular tachycardia and ventricular fibrillation could develop.

   c. Anticoagulants to reduce the hazard of embolization

   d. Procainamide, if quinidine cannot be tolerated

2. **Paroxysmal atrial fibrillation:**

   a. Digitalis—probably rapid digitalization

   b. Oxygen

   c. Procainamide is usually contraindicated because of its hypotensive effect.

   d. Vasopressors

   e. Countershock might be the first choice of many physicians.

NURSING RESPONSIBILITIES

1. Identify and document with an ECG.
2. Assess clinical state. Check vital signs.
3. If sudden in onset, notify physician at once.
4. Be alert for symptoms of coronary insufficiency (angina), shock or congestive failure.
5. Be alert for signs of toxicity of digitalis or antiarrhythmic drugs.
6. Be prepared to assist with countershock.

    Figure 10–11 presents atrial fibrillation with slow ventricular response. The P waves are absent and the base line undulates. The QRS falls very irregularly and at a very slow rate.

    Figure 10–12 presents atrial fibrillation. The P waves are absent.

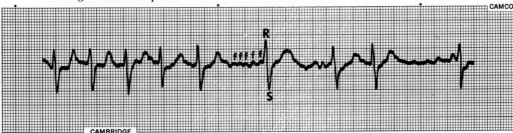

FIG. 10–12. Atrial fibrillation.

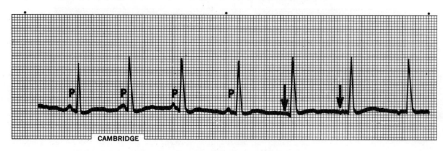

Fɪɢ. 10–13. Wandering pacemaker.

Fibrillatory waves are present at rates up to 500 per minute. Ventricular response is irregularly irregular at rates varying from 70 to 118. The QRS is normal.

Wandering Pacemaker

Wandering pacemaker is a disturbance of pacemaker function characterized by very slight variations in rhythm. The S-A node is the pacemaker of the basic rhythm. With increased vagal tone, the S-A node is suppressed. The following impulse arises in the atria. With further increase in vagal tone, the ectopic atrial focus is suppressed and the A-V node discharges an impulse. The pacemaker "wanders" back and forth from the S-A node to the A-V node.

ETIOLOGY

1. Increased vagal tone. Increased vagal tone suppresses faster pacemakers earlier than the slower ones.
2. Digitalis
3. Organic and rheumatic heart disease

CLINICAL ASPECTS

There are no signs or symptoms. The diagnosis is made with an ECG. The patient should be monitored for further signs of irritability in the atria.

ECG FINDINGS

1. Changing configuration and direction of P wave
2. Changing P-P interval
3. Slowing of rate
4. Decrease in P-R interval to less than 0.12 second

TREATMENT

None

NURSING RESPONSIBILITIES
1. Identify and document with an ECG.
2. Be alert for signs of atrial irritability.

Figure 10–13 illustrates markedly wandering pacemaker. There is a P wave before each QRS. The P wave changes in contour, height and positivity, thus indicating that the impulse is arising in the S-A node, atria, low in the atria or near the A-V node. The P-R interval becomes shorter as the impulse comes closer to the A-V node.

ATRIO-VENTRICULAR NODE

The disorders in impulse formation arising in the A-V node are premature nodal beats, nodal rhythm and nodal tachycardia.

Premature Nodal Beats (PNB)

A premature nodal beat is a heartbeat which occurs early due to a disturbance of pacemaker function. Premature nodal beats are sometimes called premature junctional beats. They arise from an ectopic focus in the A-V node. The atria are usually activated in a retrograde fashion. The ectopic focus can be high, A-V junctional, or lower nodal. Conduction to the ventricles is normal.

ETIOLOGY

See discussion of premature beats in Chapter 9.

CLINICAL ASPECTS

Diagnosis is made by an ECG. Signs or symptoms of premature nodal beats are rare, and are clinically significant only if they increase in incidence to a frequency of more than six per minute. They can be precursors of a more serious nodal arrhythmia.

ECG FINDINGS

If the ectopic focus is high in the A-V node, the P wave comes before the QRS and is inverted. The P-R interval is less than 0.12 second.

If the impulse arises in the middle of the node, the P wave is hidden in the QRS, because the atria are being activated by retrograde conduction simultaneously with the activation of the ventricles by normal conduction.

If the impulse arises in the lower portion of the node, an inverted P wave follows the QRS, because the ventricles are activated before the atria, which are activated by retrograde conduction.

The QRS is normal if ventricular conduction is normal, unless the P wave falls within the QRS, in which case the QRS may be slightly widened and slightly distorted.

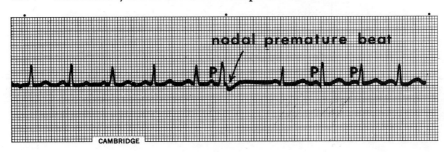

Fig. 10–14. Nodal premature beat.

The QRS of ventricular response may be absent if the premature nodal impulse reaches the ventricle in its absolute refractory period. As a rule, the QRS of the PNB is that of the basic rhythm.

The pause following a PNB is not compensatory, because the S-A node has been depolarized by retrograde conduction. Where there is no retrograde atrial depolarization, the S-A node continues its basic rhythm, the P wave occurs on time and the compensatory pause is complete.

TREATMENT

Usually no treatment is given unless more than six PNB's occur per minute. Then antiarrhythmic drugs are instituted, and attempts are made to correct electrolyte imbalance. Vasopressors are used if indicated.

NURSING RESPONSIBILITIES

1. Identify and document with an ECG.
2. Notify physician if incidence increases to six PNB's per minute.

Figure 10–14 presents premature nodal beat. The seventh R wave comes early and is followed by an inverted P wave. Conduction to the atria is retrograde from the A-V node. The R-R interval of the premature beat added to the R-R interval of the subsequent beat does not equal the sum of the R-R of two normal beats. The pause following the premature beat is not compensatory.

A-V Nodal Rhythm

A-V nodal rhythm is a disturbance of pacemaker function characterized by a slow pulse of 40–70 per minute. It is an escape rhythm in which a secondary pacemaker in the A-V node takes over by default of the S-A node. Conduction to the ventricles is normal.

ETIOLOGY

1. Depression of S-A node by vagus
2. Organic heart disease with injury to S-A node
3. Digitalis intoxication

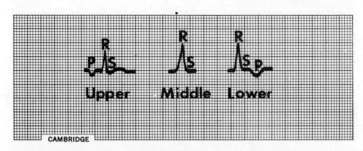

Fig. 10–15. Relationship of P wave to QRS.

CLINICAL ASPECTS

With nodal rhythm, symptoms are rare unless the rhythm takes an extremely slow rate. The diagnosis must be made by ECG.

ECG FINDINGS

There are three classic patterns of nodal rhythm with retrograde conduction to the atria. This would seem to imply that there are three potential pacemaker sites in the A-V node. The present view is that the middle nodal area probably does not possess pacemaker cells and that the relative position of the P wave to the QRS is determined by the relative speeds of retrograde conduction to the atria and antegrade conduction to the ventricles.

For the sake of convenience, the terms *upper, middle* and *lower* nodal are still used, not as a definition of pacemaker site, but as a definition of the relative position of the P wave to the QRS as indicated in Figure 10–15.

In upper nodal rhythm, an inverted P wave precedes the QRS. This rhythm has to be distinguished from coronary sinus rhythm, in which the pacemaker site is low in the atria near the opening of the coronary sinus. If the P-R interval is 0.12 second or more, the pacemaker site is assumed to be coronary sinus. If the P-R interval is less than 0.12 second, the pacemaker site is assumed to be A-V nodal.

In middle nodal (junctional) rhythm, the P wave is hidden in the QRS. In lower nodal rhythm, an inverted P wave follows the QRS. The QRS is that of the basic rhythm.

In lower nodal rhythm in which the ventricle is activated before the atria, the retrograde atrial activation wave may be sufficiently delayed so that, after activating the atria, it re-enters the A-V node and passes to the ventricles, producing another ventricular response. This mechanism is called *A-V nodal rhythm with reciprocal beats,* and may be a precursor of supraventricular tachycardia.

A nodal pacemaker may take control of the ventricles in complete A-V block. The atria remain under control of an atrial pacemaker.

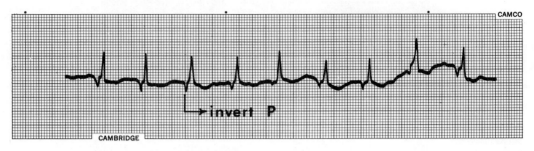

FIG. 10–16. Upper nodal rhythm.

There is dissociation of the atria and ventricles, with the atrial rate being faster than the ventricular rate.

TREATMENT

The treatment is that of the underlying disease and elimination of any known causative factors. Atropine is sometimes used for its effect on the vagus to encourage the sinus node to take over.

NURSING RESPONSIBILITIES

1. Identify and document with an ECG.
2. Watch for A-V block or development of rapid arrhythmias.
3. Withhold digitalis pending physician's instructions.
4. Assess clinical state and check vital signs.

Figure 10–16 presents upper nodal rhythm. Inverted, peaked, narrow P waves precede each QRS. The P-R interval is less than 0.12 second. Atrial and ventricular rates are both 88.

Figure 10–17 illustrates middle nodal (junctional) rhythm. The R-R intervals are regular at a rate of 78. The P waves are hidden in the QRS.

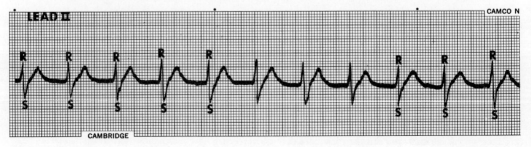

FIG. 10–17. Middle nodal (junctional) rhythm.

Nodal Tachycardia

Nodal tachycardia is a disturbance of impulse formation characterized by a rapid, regular pulse rate of 120–200. When some pathological state so enhances the automaticity of the A-V node that it exceeds that of the S-A node, then the A-V node abruptly and actively assumes the role of pacemaker. As with premature nodal beats, the impulse may be formed at high, middle or lower nodal sites.

Occasionally, but not usually, nodal tachycardia is preceded by premature nodal beats. It is usually paroxysmal in nature, though it may become the dominant rhythm. It comes under the general heading of supraventricular tachycardias, that is to say, the ectopic focus is above the common bundle. The ectopic focus stimulates the atria in retrograde fashion, and the ventricles in normal fashion. Because atria and ventricles are being controlled by the same pacemaker, the atrial and ventricular complexes bear a constant relationship to each other.

ETIOLOGY

Nodal tachycardia is a relatively rare arrhythmia. It is associated with hyperthyroidism, digitalis toxicity, potassium depletion and myocardial infarction. It can occur in normal hearts with no apparent cause.

HEMODYNAMICS

At rates over 150 there is poor ventricular filling and decreased cardiac output. The significance depends upon the underlying heart condition. It is a dangerous rhythm in coronary heart disease.

CLINICAL ASPECTS

The rapid rate is usually well tolerated, although the patient may complain of palpitation and dyspnea. In underlying heart disease, such as myocardial infarction, oppressive chest pain may appear. Signs of shock and failure may develop.

When nodal tachycardia complicates myocardial infarction, it usually has its onset several days after the acute infarction.

ECG FINDINGS

1. Rate 120–200. The pattern resembles atrial tachycardia, except that negative P waves before or after the QRS appear in lead II.
2. The P wave may be lost in the QRS. The P waves in nodal tachycardia are usually less than 0.12 second from the QRS when they precede it. However, the P-R may be longer. The QRS is that of the basic rhythm.

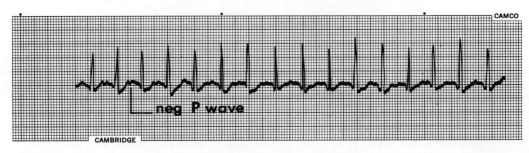

Fig. 10–18. Low nodal tachycardia.

3. In very rapid rates, the presence or absence of P waves sometimes cannot be definitely confirmed by usual ECG leads. If the QRS complexes are normal in direction and configuration in these instances, the arrhythmia is usually simply labeled "supraventricular tachycardia," perhaps with the conviction that the use of other than ordinary means to pinpoint the exact ectopic focus would be an academic exercise.

TREATMENT

The urgency for treatment is related to the degree of heart disease. It is important that the arrhythmia be abolished quickly if signs of shock or failure appear.

Carotid sinus stimulation is sometimes applied by the physician, under controlled conditions and with due regard to the possibility of inducing cardiac arrest.

Sedation, digitalis, quinidine and correction of electrolyte disturbances are tried. If cardiac failure is imminent, countershock is given.

NURSING RESPONSIBILITIES

1. Identify and document with an ECG.
2. Assess clinical state and check vital signs.
3. Notify physician immediately.
4. Administer antiarrhythmic drugs as ordered.
5. Be prepared to assist with countershock.

Figure 10–18 presents low nodal tachycardia. There is a negative P wave after each QRS. The R-R interval is regular at a rate of 150.

VENTRICLES

The disorders in impulse formation arising in the ventricles are premature ventricular contractions, ventricular tachycardia, ventricular fibrillation, idioventricular rhythm and ventricular standstill.

Premature Ventricular Contractions (PVC)

A premature ventricular contraction is a disturbance of impulse formation, characterized by a ventricular beat which comes early with relation to the basic rhythm. These premature beats are known variously as premature ventricular contractions, premature ventricular beats or ventricular extrasystoles. "Extrasystole" is a misnomer, since only one type of PVC is an "extra" beat, that is, the interpolated beat.

The impulse for the PVC arises in an irritable ectopic focus in either ventricle. The ventricles contract before the atria in response to the ectopic impulse. The atria continue to respond to S-A nodal impulse, unless there is retrograde conduction from ventricle to atria.

When a PVC occurs in a run of normal sinus rhythm, the pause following the premature beat is fully compensatory. The total time measurement of one normal beat plus one premature ventricular beat equals the time of two normal beats, because the basic impulse formation in the S-A node is not usually disturbed in the absence of retrograde conduction.

However, retrograde conduction to the atria can occur if the PVC impulse falls at the nonrefractory period of the A-V node. The S-A node then will depolarize early due to the retrograde conduction, and the compensatory pause will not be complete.

The pause following a premature ventricular contraction may be terminated by a normal sinus beat, an escape supraventricular beat or rhythm, or by a nodal escape beat or rhythm. This would be most likely to occur in sinus bradycardia or S-A block.

More than one ventricular ectopic focus may be operative. The PVC's may occur singly, in salvos, or in fixed relationship with the normal beat—bigeminy, trigeminy, and so on.

At slow rates, the PVC may be *interpolated,* with no compensatory pause, because the ventricle will have lost its refractoriness before the next normal sinus beat. This is the true *extra*systole.

PVC's usually fall early in diastole, but they may fall late, coinciding with atrial activation. A *fusion* beat may result.

Premature ventricular contractions during refractory period: The Q-T interval represents the refractory period, and the T wave represents the relative refractory. PVC's usually fall after the T wave of the previous beat. If it falls within the T wave of the previous beat, it indicates that the ectopic impulse giving rise to the premature beat has the capability of assuming the role of pacemaker in a ventricular tachycardia. The R wave of ventricular depolarization falls on the T wave of ventricular repolarization in its relative refractory period. This is often called the "R on T phenomenon."

ETIOLOGY

1. Organic heart disease
2. Coronary artery disease or infarction
3. Drugs—digitalis or quinidine
4. Electrolyte imbalance
5. May occur in normal hearts

HEMODYNAMICS

The ventricle contracts before it has a chance to fill completely. If the premature beat occurs with frequency, there is a diminution of cardiac output. The average reduction of coronary blood flow of the PVC is 12 per cent.

CLINICAL ASPECTS

The patient will probably complain of palpitation or that his heart is skipping beats. The radial pulse is irregular and the compensatory pause can be detected at the wrist or apically.

No significance need be attached to the occasional PVC in a normal heart. Where there is underlying heart disease or myocardial infarction, the occurrence of PVC's implies myocardial irritability, predisposing the individual to serious rhythm problems.

If the PVC's occur more often than six per minute, in salvos or in bigeminy, the danger of ventricular tachycardia or fibrillation is grave. Multifocal PVC's or bigeminy are often due to digitalis toxicity.

ECG FINDINGS

1. The PVC is characterized by a QRS occurring prematurely and not related to a P wave.
2. The QRS is usually wide, slurred, or notched, because conduction is through muscle and not through the Purkinje system.
3. The T wave of repolarization is opposite in direction to the main deflection of the QRS (discordant).
4. If more than one ectopic focus is operative, the QRS of the premature beats will not be identical.
5. If the ectopic focus is in the right ventricle, depolarization is from the right to the left—toward the positive left-arm electrode of lead I. The QRS is therefore positive in deflection, and the T wave negative in lead I.
6. If the ectopic focus is in the left ventricle, depolarization is from left to right—away from the positive left-arm electrode in lead I. The QRS is therefore negative in deflection, and the T wave positive in lead I.

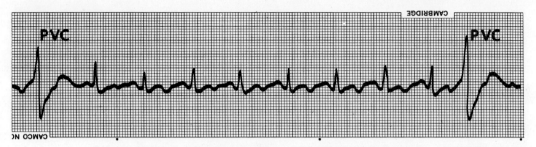

FIG. 10–19. Occasional premature ventricular contractions.

7. The R-R of the normal beat added to the R-R of the premature beat equal two R-R's of the basic rhythm (compensatory pause).
8. In an interpolated PVC, the QRS of the premature beat is injected between two normally timed beats.
9. In the fusion beat in which atria and ventricles are stimulated simultaneously, the first part of the QRS is bizarre due to the ectopic focus, and the terminal portion is normal due to normal conduction through the bundle, or vice versa.
10. In PVC with retrograde atrial conduction, the compensatory pause is not complete and the P wave is inverted in lead II.
11. Premature ventricular contractions may occur as interruptions of other arrhythmias, such as atrial fibrillation.

TREATMENT

1. Lidocaine
2. Sedation
3. Discontinuation of suspect drugs such as digitalis
4. Quinidine
5. Procainamide
6. Dilantin—especially if the disorder is digitalis-induced.
7. Potassium replacement

NURSING RESPONSIBILITIES

1. Identify and document with an ECG.
2. Record time of onset and frequency.
3. Notify physician if symptoms arise or frequency increases.
4. Give sedation as indicated if ordered.
5. Give antiarrhythmic drugs as ordered.
6. Question standing orders for digitalis.

Figure 10–19 displays two premature ventricular beats, as marked. A 69-year-old man with no previous illness was admitted with severe

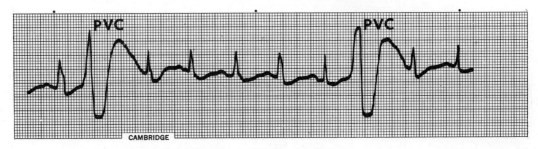

Fig. 10–20. Frequent premature ventricular contractions.

chest pain two days before this strip was run. Routine laboratory work and follow-up revealed mild diabetes. Acute anterior infarction was confirmed by a full ECG. The patient was placed on anticoagulants.

As shown in Figure 10–19, the patient began to have occasional premature ventricular beats. The patient was not aware of the PVC's and there was no drop in blood pressure. Oral quinidine controlled this very mild arrhythmia, and the patient went on to convalescence.

In Figure 10–20 there are two PVC's in a 6-inch strip (representing 6 seconds), characterized by absent P waves, broad QRS and discordant T wave. If the rate of occurrence were constant, there would be 20 PVC's per minute. The rate of the basic rhythm is about 90. The percentage of relatively inefficient beats per minute is therefore quite high.

Figure 10–21 presents ventricular bigeminy. Normal and abnormal beats are paired. The abnormal beat is not preceded by a P wave, the QRS is wide and the T wave is discordant.

Figure 10–22 presents ventricular trigeminy. Two normal beats alternate with one abnormal. The QRS of the abnormal beat is wide and not preceded by a P wave. The T wave is discordant. First degree A-V block is also present, as evidenced by the prolonged P-R interval.

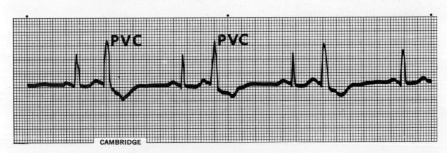

Fig. 10–21. Ventricular bigeminy.

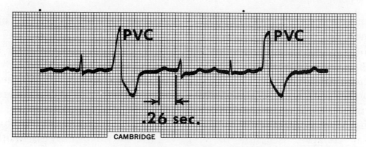

Fig. 10–22. Ventricular trigeminy.

Ventricular Tachycardia

Ventricular tachycardia is a disturbance of impulse formation characterized by a rapid, almost regular, ventricular rate of 150–200, independent of atrial activity. The impulse for this rapid arrhythmia arises in a ventricular ectopic focus. It is often preceded by one or more premature ventricular contractions. It is usually unifocal.

A paroxysm of ventricular tachycardia is composed of six or more premature ventricular beats in rapid succession. It may become the dominant rhythm.

ETIOLOGY

1. Myocardial infarction
2. Hypertension
3. Myocarditis
4. Heart failure
5. Cardiac injuries such as stabbings or contusions
6. Cardiac surgery, catheterization, or angiography
7. Drugs—Adrenalin, quinidine, digitalis, procainamide
8. Anesthetic agents—chloroform or cyclopropane, especially if used with Adrenalin

HEMODYNAMICS

Ventricular tachycardia may or may not cause severe hemodynamic disturbances.

When the ectopic focus triggering the ventricular contractions is near the apex, the wave of muscle contraction starts near the apex, and the whole ventricular response closely resembles the normal.

When the ectopic focus is near the base of the heart, the muscle contraction starts near the base of the heart and pushes the blood towards the apex, away from the outflow tract. The blood is then pushed back in the direction of the outflow tract. By the time the blood reaches the semilunar valves, normal output is hindered by the narrowing of the outflow tract in systole.

The asynchronous atrial and ventricular activity results in poor atrial emptying, back pressure and poor ventricular filling.

The cardiac output in ventricular tachycardia is diminished in proportion as the ventricular rate increases, qualified by the degree of abnormality of the ventricular contractions.

The diminished cardiac output may result in hypotension, peripheral vascular collapse, ischemia of vital organs and coronary ischemia or infarction. If coronary infarction is already present, the infarction may spread. Ventricular tachycardia may reduce coronary blood flow by 60 per cent or more.

CLINICAL ASPECTS

The patient may complain of a thumping sensation in head or chest. The pulse may run from 100 to 200 per minute and be slightly irregular. The patient may be pale, perspire profusely, be short of breath, and have substernal pain. The blood pressure may disappear, the patient may become cyanotic and lose consciousness, and all the signs of shock and failure may be present.

Ventricular tachycardia may stop spontaneously after a short run, but it may evolve into ventricular fibrillation or asystole. Ventricular tachycardia in the patient with a coronary infarction is a grave emergency.

ECG FINDINGS

1. P waves may follow the QRS due to retrograde atrial conduction, but they are usually hidden in the larger complex, or there may be an independent sinus P.
2. QRS complexes at a rapid rate usually have the same configuration as the premature ventricular beats which may have preceded the onset. If more than one ectopic focus is operative, the QRS will carry the configuration of the ectopic focus for the individual beat.
3. The ectopic foci may alternate beat for beat, and the QRS will alternate in direction and configuration. Bidirectional ventricular tachycardia may really be junctional with alternating conducting pathways, capture and fusion. This mechanism creates competitive muscular forces in the ventricles which greatly impede ventricular emptying.
4. The QRS is wider than 0.12 second. At rapid rates, the S-T segment and T waves are difficult to identify and appear as a continuum of the QRS.

TREATMENT

1. Lidocaine
2. Countershock

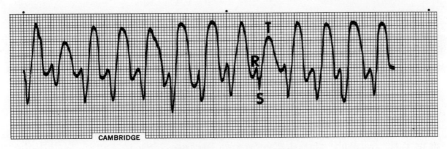

FIG. 10–23. Ventricular tachycardia.

3. Relief of anxiety—opiates, barbiturates
4. Quinidine or procainamide to suppress myocardial irritability
5. Potassium replacement if indicated
6. Dilantin, if arrhythmia is digitalis-induced. *Caution:* Cardiac arrests have followed the use of dilantin.
7. Vasopressors

NURSING RESPONSIBILITIES
1. Identify and document with an ECG. Keep write-out operating continuously.
2. Sound physician alarm.
3. Assess clinical state and check vital signs continuously.
4. Administer antiarrhythmic drugs, or prepare them for administration.
5. Assist with countershock.
6. Monitor for recurrence.

Figure 10–23 presents ventricular tachycardia. There are no discernible P waves. The QRS complexes are those of the premature ventricular contraction. They are bizarre and vary somewhat in configuration. The R-R is almost regular at a rate of 140.

Figure 10–24 presents ventricular flutter, which is an advanced form of ventricular tachycardia often associated with digitalis intoxication and

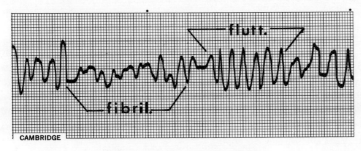

FIG. 10–24. Ventricular flutter.

coronary thrombosis. T waves, P waves and iso-electric lines are absent. QRS complexes have little resemblance to normal, and are wide and uniform-appearing at a rate of 300 plus.

Ventricular Fibrillation

Ventricular fibrillation is a catastrophic arrhythmia in which the ventricular muscles lose their ability to contract and function as a unit. Repetitive stimuli from an ectopic ventricular pacemaker are discharged at a rate so rapid that the ventricles are not able to respond, and the normal forceful muscular contraction is replaced by irregular, rapid, uncoordinated twitching. Because the ventricles do not pump, circulation ceases. If not reversed in a very few minutes, the vital organs are irreversibly damaged and death comes quickly.

ETIOLOGY
1. Coronary ischemia or occlusion
2. Anesthetic agents
3. Accidental electrocution
4. Penetrating wounds of the heart
5. Cardiac surgery, catheterization or cardio-angiography
6. Drugs—digitalis, quinidine, procainamide
7. Hypoxia:
    a. Pulmonary edema
    b. Obstruction to airway
    c. Strangulation
    d. Chronic pulmonary disease

CLINICAL ASPECTS FROM TIME OF ONSET
1. 3-4 seconds—weakness, dizziness
2. 10-20 seconds—syncope, convulsion, absence of heart sounds, absence of pulse, absence of blood pressure
3. 40-50 seconds—incontinence, apnea, pallor, dilated pupils, agonal respirations
4. 4 minutes—death can occur, but patients have been resuscitated after longer periods.

The point of no return in ventricular fibrillation depends upon the metabolic state of myocardium when fibrillation began. In the laboratory, animals under anesthesia are made to fibrillate by an electrical stimulus. If the animal has been well oxygenated and is perfusing well, the induced fibrillation can be readily converted to normal sinus rhythm by countershock. The poorer the perfusion and oxygenation, the less likelihood that defibrillation can be accomplished.

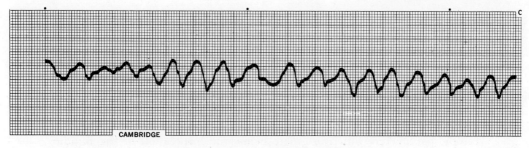

Fig. 10–25. Ventricular fibrillation.

ECG FINDINGS

Ventricular fibrillation is often preceded by paroxysmal ventricular tachycardia. It is usually preceded by multifocal premature ventricular beats. The QRS becomes wider and more aberrant. At the rate of 175-220 per minute, the QRS and T fuse. There is no iso-electric line. The complex becomes more irregular and distorted. The amplitude decreases to an undulating base line, ending in the straight line of cardiac standstill.

TREATMENT

When ventricular fibrillation occurs, countershock must be used as soon as possible. If a cardioverter is not available, mouth-to-mouth breathing or other forms of assisted respiration and external cardiac massage must be started at once, following up with full-scale cardiac resuscitation procedure as discussed in Chapter 7 under Cardiac Arrest.

NURSING RESPONSIBILITIES

1. Identify and document with an ECG. In those monitors with automatic write-out and alarm systems, the write-out will activate itself. Keep the write-out in continuous operation.
2. Sound alarm for cardiac resuscitation team.
3. Notify physician at once.
4. When time available to personnel permits, notify family of patient's critical condition.
5. Help the family and the patient to meet the requirements of their religious beliefs. Every effort should be made to maintain informative and sympathetic communication with the patient's family during the resuscitation procedure.

In ventricular fibrillation, shown in Figure 10–25, it is impossible to identify any wave forms, segments or intervals. Totally irregular waves, varying in configuration, width and amplitude, appear, and there is no iso-electric line.

Idioventricular Rhythm

Idioventricular rhythm is a disturbance of pacemaker function characterized by a slow pulse of 30–35. The failure or blocking of the S-A node and the A-V node results in a ventricular ectopic pacemaker taking over at its own slow rhythmicity.

In complete heart block, some authorities call the ventricular pacemaker which takes over "idioventricular," regardless of the site of the ventricular ectopic focus. Others reserve the term for those ventricular ectopic pacemakers which originate below the bifurcation of the bundle of His, in spite of the fact that part of the common bundle is anatomically a ventricular structure.

If the ectopic focus arises above the bifurcation, ventricular conduction may be normal and have a faster rate than those arising below the bifurcation.

If the ectopic focus is in the left bundle branch, the pattern of the QRS will be that of right bundle branch block.

If the ectopic focus is in the right bundle branch, the QRS will be that of left bundle branch block.

When the ectopic focus is in the Purkinje fibers or in ventricular muscle, ventricular conduction is aberrant, and the rate is in the range of 20–30.

There is usually no retrograde conduction to the atria. Atrial activity is independent of ventricular activity and under control of a supraventricular pacemaker if one is operative.

There is usually a prolonged pause before the ventricular pacemaker takes over. This is called the "pre-automatic" pause.

ETIOLOGY

1. Severe organic heart disease
2. Digitalis intoxication

CLINICAL ASPECTS

Where the idioventricular rhythm arises suddenly as a consequence of periodic and sudden changes from normal A-V conduction or partial A-V block to complete A-V block, the dramatic decrease in cardiac output may result in Adams-Stokes attack, which may terminate in death.

If complete A-V block is established, and idioventricular rhythm is established, compatibility with life depends upon the ventricular rate. The rate of idioventricular rhythm is not responsive to exercise. Even those ventricular rates which may sustain life will precipitate syncope and Adams-Stokes attack when metabolic demands are increased. In such instances, the artificial pacemaker is used.

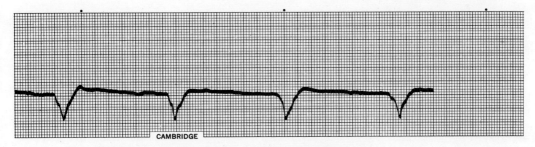
CAMBRIDGE

Fig. 10–26. Idioventricular rhythm.

ECG FINDINGS
1. If the S-A node is active, P waves occur with no fixed relationship to the QRS.
2. If the ectopic focus is above the bifurcation of the bundle of His, the QRS is normal at a rate of 30-40.
3. If the ectopic focus is in the bundle branches, the QRS is wide and bizarre at a rate of 20-30.

TREATMENT
1. Artificial pacemaker
2. No antiarrhythmic drugs, since they may depress the ectopic pacemaker to the point of asystole
3. Digitalis to increase force of contraction only if complete A-V block is present
4. Vasopressors
5. Defibrillation if fibrillation occurs

NURSING RESPONSIBILITIES
1. Identify and document with an ECG.
2. Notify physician if arrhythmia occurs suddenly.
3. Be prepared for all-out emergency measures.

Figure 10–26 presents idioventricular rhythm. There is no evidence of atrial activity. Wide ventricular complexes appear at a slow rate.

Ventricular Standstill
Current usage defines cardiac arrest as the sudden, unexpected cessation of effective heartbeat. Ventricular standstill is one of the mechanisms of cardiac arrest. Ventricular fibrillation is the other.

Ventricular standstill can manifest itself as **ventricular asystole** or as **total asystole.**

Ventricular asystole results when atrial stimulation is blocked from

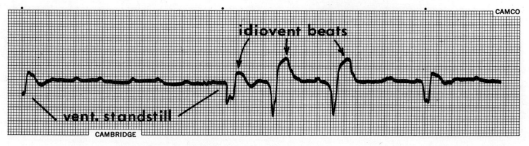

FIG. 10–27. Ventricular standstill with atrial activity.

the ventricles by the existence of A-V block when there is absence of a ventricular pacemaker. This is particularly true if the A-V block is sudden in onset.

ETIOLOGY

1. Organic heart disease
2. May follow open-heart surgery
3. Drugs which depress ventricular pacemaker: digitalis, quinidine, procainamide
4. Vagal stimulation

ECG FINDINGS

P waves are present and continue to be normal for a time after ventricular activity ceases. The QRS is totally absent. If not reversed, P waves of atrial activity disappear and the ECG consists of a slightly undulating or straight line.

CLINICAL ASPECTS

The symptoms are loss of consciousness and possible convulsion, pallor, absence of pulse, and Cheyne-Stokes respirations. An Adams-Stokes attack may abort itself in 20 seconds. Recovery is rare after 60 seconds.

TREATMENT

1. Sharp blow to chest over heart
2. Cardiac massage
3. Assisted respiration
4. Intracardiac Adrenalin
5. Emergency artificial pacemaking—external or transthoracic needle electrode
6. Preventive treatment is that of the underlying block. In the face of progressing block following acute myocardial infarction, a transvenous pacemaker electrode catheter may be positioned for stand-by or demand pacing.

Figure 10–27 presents ventricular standstill, due to complete A-V

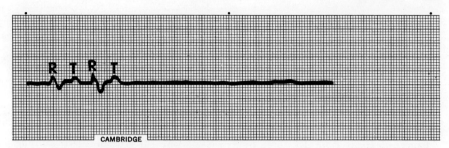

FIG. 10–28. Total asystole preceded by idioventricular rhythm.

block, with atrial activity. At the beginning of this strip is a series of P waves of atrial activity, with no ventricular response (representing ventricular standstill), followed by a few idioventricular beats.

Total asystole results from sinus standstill, A-V standstill and absence of tertiary pacemaker in the ventricles.

ETIOLOGY

1. Depression of electrical activity due to shock
2. Congestive failure
3. Anoxia
4. Electrolyte imbalance
5. Circulatory failure

ECG FINDINGS

1. P waves of atrial activity are absent.
2. Broad, slurred QRS of idioventricular beats may continue for a short time after cessation of atrial activity.
3. If not reversed, the idioventricular rhythm fades out into a slightly undulating or straight line.

CLINICAL ASPECTS

The signs and symptoms of total asystole are those of the underlying shock or circulatory failure and of cardiac arrest. The prognosis is poor due to underlying disease. Resuscitative procedure and emergency pacemaking may be attempted.

The differentiation between standstill and fibrillation can only be made by ECG. The treatment for standstill is pacemaking; the treatment for fibrillation is defibrillation.

Figure 10–28 presents total asystole preceded by idioventricular rhythm. This strip begins with three idioventricular beats showing no evidence of atrial activity. This is followed by a slightly undulating straight line, representing total asystole.

REFERENCES AND BIBLIOGRAPHY

Bernreiter, M.: Electrocardiography. ed. 2. Philadelphia, J. B. Lippincott, 1963.

Burch, T., and Winsor, T.: A Primer of Electrocardiography. ed. 5. Philadelphia, Lea & Febiger, 1966.

Corday, E., and Irving, D. W.: Disturbances of Heart Rate, Rhythm, and Conduction. ed. 2. W. B. Saunders, 1962.

Friedberg, C. K.: Diseases of the Heart. ed. 3. Philadelphia, W. B. Saunders, 1966.

Goldman, M. J.: Principles of Clinical Electrocardiography. ed. 6. Los Altos, California, Lange Medical Publications, 1967.

Guyton, A. C.: Textbook of Medical Physiology. ed. 3. Philadelphia, W. B. Saunders, 1968.

Jude, J. R., and Elam, J. O.: Fundamentals of Cardio-Pulmonary Resuscitation. Philadelphia, F. A. Davis, 1965.

Ritota, M.: Diagnostic Electrocardiography. Philadelphia, J. B. Lippincott, 1969.

Schaub, R.: Fundamentals of Clinical Electrocardiography. Switzerland, Documenta Geigy, Ardsley, N.Y., 1966.

Wood, P.: Diseases of the Heart and Circulation. ed. 3. Philadelphia, J. B. Lippincott, 1968.

11 CARDIAC ARRHYTHMIAS: DISORDERS OF IMPULSE CONDUCTION

In normal sinus rhythm, the electrical impulse which originates in the S-A node is conducted throughout the heart in a timed, orderly sequence. This chapter discusses the disorders resulting from disturbances in impulse conduction. The material is presented according to the sites at which these disorders originate, namely the S-A node, the atria, the A-V node, the bundle branches and the Purkinje system.

SINO-ATRIAL BLOCK

S-A block is a disturbance of conduction from the S-A node, in which one or more heartbeats are "skipped."

The impulse is initiated normally in the S-A node, but a pathological state in or surrounding the S-A node prevents transmission of the impulse to the atria. The atria do not depolarize, and this results in atrial standstill.

The standstill may terminate in a normal sinus rhythm. If the block is intermittent, every other sinus impulse may be conducted normally, giving the block the clinical appearance of sinus bradycardia.

If the S-A block is complete, the atrial standstill may terminate in nodal escape rhythm.

ETIOLOGY
1. Drugs—digitalis, quinidine, Neo-Synephrine
2. Hyperkalemia
3. Vagal stimulants
4. Anesthetic agents
5. Cerebral lesions
6. Organic disease in or around the S-A node
7. Atrial infarction

151

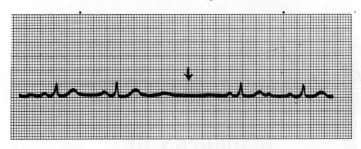

FIG. 11–1. Sino-atrial block.

CLINICAL ASPECTS

With long or frequent pauses, the patient may complain of faintness, dizziness, or even have Adams-Stokes syncope. Death may occur from cardiac standstill if other pacemakers do not take over when the S-A node defaults for too long a period.

S-A block is classified as first, second and third degree, in terms of increasing block.

ECG FINDINGS

1. **First degree** is difficult to distinguish in the ECG.
2. **Second degree** occurs in three forms:
   a. Slow heart rate abruptly doubles after change of body position or exercise. This is 2:1 S-A block.
   b. Wenckebach type: If only one impulse has been blocked, the P-P interval, including a blocked S-A impulse, is less than twice the P-P interval preceding it. The P-P interval following the dropped beat is longer than the P-P interval preceding it. There is progressive shortening of the P-P intervals up to the pause.
   c. There are occasional blocked impulses with no preliminary changes in conduction time.
3. **Third degree** cannot be distinguished from sinus arrest.

Basically, in S-A block there is a prolonged pause between two normal P-QRS-T cycles. The pauses are doubles or other multiples of the R-R intervals of the basic rhythm.

TREATMENT

1. Stop incriminated drugs.
2. The following drugs may be given:
   a. Ephedrine
   b. Isuprel
   c. Atropine

NURSING RESPONSIBILITIES
1. Identify and document with an ECG.
2. Assess clinical state and check vital signs.
3. Notify physician.
4. Reaffirm orders for digitalis or quinidine.
5. Watch for escape rhythms.

Figure 11–1 demonstrates S-A block. It shows one dropped P-QRS-T in a run of normal sinus rhythm. The R-R interval covering the dropped beat is exactly double the R-R interval of the normal beats.

INTRA-ATRIAL BLOCK

Intra-atrial block is a prolongation of the transmission time of the impulse conduction through atrial muscle. It is seen in those heart conditions which damage or enlarge atrial muscle, for example mitral heart disease. The slowed conduction in the atria manifests itself in the ECG in changes in the P wave, which may become slurred, notched and prolonged beyond 0.10 second.

ATRIO-VENTRICULAR NODE

The disorders in impulse conduction arising in the A-V node are A-V dissociation, interference dissociation, fusion beats, and heart block.

A-V Dissociation Without A-V Block

A-V dissociation without A-V block exists if, for one or more beats, the atria and ventricles are controlled by different pacemakers in the absence of antegrade block, in the presence of retrograde block, with an idioventricular pacemaker rate of less than 150.

In the most common form, impulse formation in the S-A node is slowed by depression. The A-V node then takes over the role of pacemaker for the ventricles by right of its now faster automatic rate. While there is no antegrade block, the sinus impulse reaches the A-V node when it has been made refractory by its own impulse formation. Because there is no retrograde conduction, the S-A node is not depolarized by the A-V nodal impulse, and the S-A node continues to activate the atria.

Because the ventricular pacemaker is faster, there are more QRS complexes than P waves in the ECG. As the atria and ventricles respond, each to its own distinct pacemaker, it sometimes happens that both pacemakers discharge simultaneously; thus the P wave and QRS fall simultaneously. The P wave is either buried in the QRS or fuses with it, deforming its shape. This is called a "fusion beat."

Occasionally, A-V dissociation is not complete. An occasional S-A nodal impulse reaches the A-V node in its nonrefractory state and is conducted to the ventricles. The ventricular response to this impulse is called a *capture beat*. A-V dissociation with interference beats is called *interference dissociation* or *incomplete dissociation*.

In some instances the ventricular pacemaker is not in the A-V node, but in the ventricle itself. Usually the lower (anatomically) pacemaker is only slightly faster than the atrial pacemaker. However, it can be much faster than the atrial pacemaker if the lower pacemaker's automaticity has been enhanced by some factor.

ETIOLOGY IN ORDER OF FREQUENCY
1. Digitalis intoxication, especially when given with diuretics
2. Coronary artery disease
3. Cerebral vascular accidents
4. Rheumatic fever
5. Quinidine intoxication
6. Cardiac catheterization
7. Pulmonary embolization

TREATMENT
1. Sometimes none because of the transcience of the condition
2. Discontinue incriminated drugs.
3. Potassium replacement, if indicated
4. Atropine may restore normal sinus rhythm.

Atrio-Ventricular Block
A-V block is a delay or interruption of electrical impulse through the A-V node, due to:

1. Prolongation of the refractory phase of the A-V node
2. Diminished strength of the impulse when it reaches the A-V node. A-V block is classified as first, second and third degree in terms of increasing severity.
   Any degree of A-V block may be transient, recurrent or permanent.

ETIOLOGY
1. Organic heart disease
2. Rheumatic heart disease
3. Infectious diseases, probably due to toxic effect on the A-V node, and probably self-limited: diphtheria, measles, mumps, viruses, bacterial endocarditis, pneumonia
4. Drugs which depress A-V node—quinidine, procainamide
5. Digitalis, by direct inhibition of A-V node and bundle, and by vagal action
6. Septal defects—usually in first degree block
7. Coronary artery disease

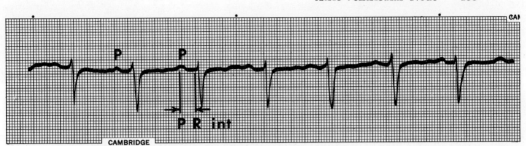

Fig. 11-2. First degree heart block.

8. Aortic stenosis—usually in third degree block
9. Luetic heart disease
10. Neoplasms of heart
11. Trauma to A-V node in heart surgery
12. Myocardial ischemia—decreased blood supply to A-V node and bundle (may persist, but normal sinus rhythm may return spontaneously after weeks.)
13. Hypoxia from anesthesia, embolization, shock, coronary occlusion or chronic pulmonary disease

First Degree Atrio-Ventricular Block

In first degree block, transmission time of impulse to and though the A-V node is prolonged. The atria contract normally, but ventricular response is slightly delayed. It is more common than second or third degree block.

CLINICAL ASPECTS

There are usually no symptoms. The diagnosis is made by ECG. Cardiac output is not affected.

ECG FINDINGS

1. P waves are regular, followed by a normal QRS.
2. The P-R interval is longer than 0.20 second.

TREATMENT

1. Watchful waiting
2. Stop suspect drugs, such as digitalis or quinidine.

NURSING RESPONSIBILITY

1. Identify and document with an ECG.
2. Measure P-R interval frequently and watch for further prolongation.

Figure 11-2 presents first degree heart block. Atrial and ventricular rates are identical at approximately 62. Normal P waves are followed by a normal QRS. The P-R interval is prolonged to 0.26 (normal is 0.20) second. This, therefore, is first degree A-V block.

Second Degree Atrio-Ventricular Block

In second degree A-V block there is an occasional blocking out of impulse at the A-V node. The atria are normally activated, but the impulse is not conducted through the A-V node to the ventricles for occasional or even alternate beats. The causes are the same for all degrees and types of A-V block. It occurs rather frequently after posterior infarction. Second degree, or partial A-V block, occurs in two distinct forms:

1. **Wenckebach, (Mobitz type 1):** The relative refractory period of the A-V node is prolonged. There is progressive lengthening of the P-R interval for successive beats, until one P wave is not followed by a QRS. The P-R interval following the pause is shorter, and the sequence repeats itself. There may or may not be some prolongation of P-R intervals for all beats in the sequence.

   The Wenckebach type of block is usually transient and rarely associated with Adams-Stokes attacks. Characteristically, 1:1 conduction can be restored by any factor which increases the atrial rate, such as exercise or atropine. Vagal stimulation, such as carotid sinus massage, will slow the atrial rate and increase the severity of the block.

2. **Mobitz type 2:** In mild forms, there is no prolongation of the P-R interval. In severe forms, there is a constant prolongation of the P-R interval. The absolute refractory period of the A-V node is prolonged. Atrial activation is normal, but there is failure to conduct the stimulus through the A-V node, so that an occasional, or even every second, third, fourth, or fifth impulse fails to reach the ventricles. The ratio of P waves to the QRS may be constant, but may vary from 2:1, 3:1, 4:1, 5:1, and so forth.

   Mobitz type 2 block is persistent, though there may be remissions. There may be sudden onset of complete block with cardiac arrest. In contrast with Wenckebach, vagal stimulation will reduce the degree of block, and increasing the atrial rate will increase the degree of block. While Wenckebach block may revert to normal with bed rest, a stand-by pacemaker is imperative in Mobitz type 2.

NURSING RESPONSIBILITIES

1. Identify and document with an ECG.
2. Watch for prolongation of P-R and progression of block.
3. Reaffirm any orders for digitalis or antiarrhythmic drugs.
4. If block suddenly progresses to third degree, notify the physician at once. Be alert for Adams-Stokes seizure. Be prepared to start artificial pacemaking.

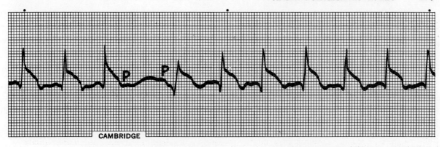

CAMBRIDGE

Fɪɢ. 11–3. Second degree A-V block, Mobitz type 2.

Figure 11–3 presents second degree A-V block, Mobitz type 2. In a run of normal sinus rhythm, only one P wave appears which is not followed by a QRS. Also present is the acute infarction pattern of S-T elevation and T wave inversion.

Figure 11–4 presents second degree block, Wenckebach type. The first P-R interval is 0.40 second. The second P-R interval prolongs to 0.54 second. The third P wave is not followed by a QRS; there is no ventricular response since the impulse has not been conducted through the A-V node. The ensuing pause allows the A-V node to recover. The P-R interval following the pause returns to 0.40 second, and the cycle repeats itself.

Third Degree Atrio-Ventricular Block

In third degree A-V block, there is no conduction from the atria to the ventricles. Each contracts independently of the other and at its own rate. There is usually no retrograde conduction.

CLINICAL ASPECTS

Cardiac output is reduced when ventricular rate is below 40. Systolic pressure is elevated, with wide pulse pressure. Inter-atrial pressure is increased.

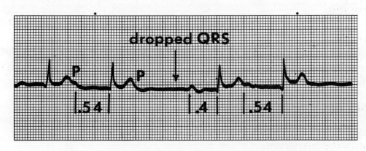

Fɪɢ. 11–4. Second degree block, Wenckebach type.

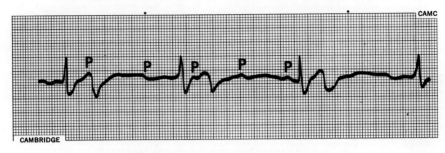

FIG. 11–5. Third degree A-V block.

The patient may complain of fatigue on exertion, angina, palpitation, and awareness of heartbeat. The pulse rate is 40 or less. There may or may not be syncope.

In third degree block, especially with sudden onset, asystole and syncope, with or without convulsions, may occur. This is the Adams-Stokes syndrome. It may terminate in 20 seconds, if an adequate idioventricular rhythm establishes itself. Recovery is rare after 60 seconds.

ECG FINDINGS

1. P waves and QRS have no fixed relationship. P waves occur more often than the QRS. P-R intervals change constantly.
2. P-P interval is regular.
3. R-R interval is regular at a rate of 40 or less.
4. QRS may or may not be abnormal in contour.
5. The ventricular pacemaker may be unstable, and ventricular asystole may develop, indicated by a series of P waves followed by no QRS complexes.

TREATMENT

1. Pacemaker
2. Isuprel
3. Atropine
4. No quinidine or procainamide because they depress the ventricular pacemaker
5. Unlike first and second degree blocks, in which digitalis is relatively contraindicated, digitalis can be used in complete block if signs of failure appear.

NURSING RESPONSIBILITIES

1. Identify and document with an ECG.
2. Notify the physician.

3. Be prepared to assist the pacemaker.
4. In asystole, a hard, sharp blow with the clenched fist to the anterior chest wall may start the heart beating. If this fails, turn on the stand-by pacemaker. If this fails, institute full-scale cardiopulmonary resuscitation.

Figure 11–5 presents third degree A-V block. Third degree A-V block is known as *complete heart block,* a type of *A-V dissociation.* There is no fixed relationship of P to QRS, indicating that the atria and ventricles are contracting independently of each other. The P-R interval varies constantly. The ventricular rate is less than 35. The atrial rate is 83.

BUNDLE BRANCH BLOCK

Bundle branch block is delay or block of the electrical impulse through either the left or right branch of the common bundle. In some instances it occurs bilaterally. The block may be complete or incomplete, and temporary or permanent.

There is a normal sinus pacemaker. Atrial and A-V nodal conduction are normal. The electrical impulse passes down the healthy bundle branch in normal fashion to stimulate the ventricle it supplies. In order for the opposite ventricle to be stimulated, the impulse must pass across the septum. When it reaches the opposite ventricle, the electrical impulse is carried by muscle rather than conductive tissue. Because electrical stimulation to one ventricle is delayed, the ventricles are stimulated asynchronously.

ETIOLOGY
1. Coronary infarction, old or fresh
2. Aortic valve disease
3. Infectious diseases
4. Quinidine, procainamide
5. Uremia—due to disturbance of calcium and potassium
6. Hyperkalemia
7. Fibrosis

CLINICAL ASPECTS
The symptoms are those of the underlying heart disease. This is an ECG diagnosis, though widely split heart sounds may suggest bundle branch block.

The implications of left bundle branch block are more serious than right bundle branch block, since it usually occurs in more serious heart conditions.

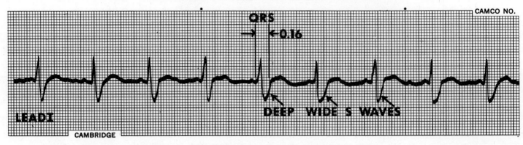

FIG. 11–6. Complete right bundle branch block.

ECG FINDINGS

Though findings of bundle branch block are evident in lead II (the usual monitor lead), it is impossible to determine in lead II which branch is involved. This can be done in lead I, in which the positive electrode is on the left arm and the negative electrode on the right arm. All the following apply to lead I.

A. **Right bundle branch block:**
1. Normal P wave
2. Wide, slurred, notched QRS
3. QRS duration greater than 0.12 second
4. Major deflection of QRS is down
5. T wave is up
6. Deep S wave

B. **Left bundle branch block:**
1. Normal P wave
2. Wide, slurred, notched QRS
3. QRS greater than 0.12 second
4. Major deflection of QRS is up
5. T wave is down
6. Q may be very small, or even absent

C. **Incomplete bundle branch block:**
The findings for left or right are as above, but the duration of the QRS is less than 0.12 second.

D. **Bilateral bundle branch block is inferred in:**
1. Right bundle branch block with left axis
2. Right or left bundle branch block with prolonged P-R time
3. Very wide QRS—greater than 0.14 second
4. Alternating bundle branch blocks

NURSING RESPONSIBILITIES

1. Identify and document with an ECG.
2. Notify the physician if the block is sudden in onset.

Figure 11–6 presents complete right bundle branch block. The QRS is

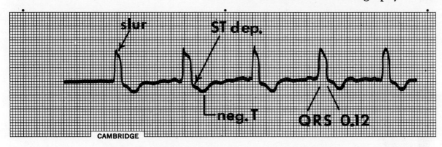

FIG. 11–7. Complete left bundle branch block.

0.16 second. There is a deep, wide S wave. The T wave is up. This is a lead I recording.

Figure 11–7 presents complete left bundle branch block. The QRS is 0.12 second and slurred. The S-T segment is depressed and the T wave is inverted. This is a lead I recording.

PURKINJE NETWORK
Arborization

Arborization block is delay or interruption of impulse transmission beyond the bundle branches in the Purkinje network. It is revealed in the ECG by a slurred QRS, prolonged beyond 0.12 second, and of low amplitude. It is generally regarded as an unfavorable prognostic sign in myocardial infarction.

REFERENCES AND BIBLIOGRAPHY

Bernreiter, M.: Electrocardiography. ed. 2. Philadelphia, J. B. Lippincott, 1963.

Burch, T., and Winsor, T.: A Primer of Electrocardiography, ed. 5. Philadelphia, Lea & Febiger, 1966.

Corday, E., and Irving, D. W.: Disturbances of Heart Rate, Rhythm and Conduction. ed. 2. Philadelphia, W. B. Saunders, 1962.

Friedberg, C. K.: Diseases of the Heart. ed. 3. Philadelphia, W. B. Saunders, 1966.

Goldman, M. J.: Principles of Clinical Electrocardiography. ed. 6. Los Altos, California, Lange Medical Publications, 1967.

Guyton, A. C.: Textbook of Medical Physiology. ed. 3. Philadelphia, W. B. Saunders, 1968.

Hurst, J. W., and Logue, R. R.: The Heart. New York, McGraw-Hill, 1966.

Jude, J. R., and Elam, J. O.: Fundamentals of Cardio-Pulmonary Resuscitation. Philadelphia, F. A. Davis, 1965.

Ritota, M.: Diagnostic Electrocardiography. Philadelphia, J. B. Lippincott, 1969.

Schaub, R.: Fundamentals of Clinical Electrocardiography. Switzerland, Documenta Geigy, 1966.

Stock, J. P. P.: Diagnosis and Treatment of Cardiac Arrhythmias. New York, Appleton-Century-Crofts, 1969.

Wood, P.: Diseases of the Heart and Circulation. ed. 3. Philadelphia, J. B. Lippincott, 1968.

12 CARE OF THE PATIENT WITH A PACEMAKER

Artificial pacing of the heart is indicated when cardiac output is insufficient to maintain adequate cerebral perfusion. The external pacemaker is designed to provide short-term pacing on an emergency basis in cardiac arrest or heart block. Heart block as a complication of myocardial infarction is usually transient. The object of artificial pacing is to maintain the ventricular rate until sinus rhythm returns spontaneously.

Emergency pacing with the external pacemaker is painful. If prolonged, the patient may suffer burns on the chest from the high voltage electrical stimulation.

TEMPORARY ENDOCARDIAL PACING

Temporary endocardial pacing involves passing a transvenous electrode to the right ventricle. The pacing catheter may be introduced through the jugular, basilic or femoral vein.

Direct pacing on a continuous or demand basis replaces painful external pacing and is indicated in:

1. High-degree A-V block complicating acute myocardial infarction
2. Complete heart block
3. Sinus arrest
4. Sinus bradycardia
5. Heart block during or after cardiac surgery

The pacing catheter is bipolar or unipolar and approximately 125 cm. in length. Under local anesthesia the catheter is usually inserted through the external jugular vein. It is then advanced and positioned in the apex

162

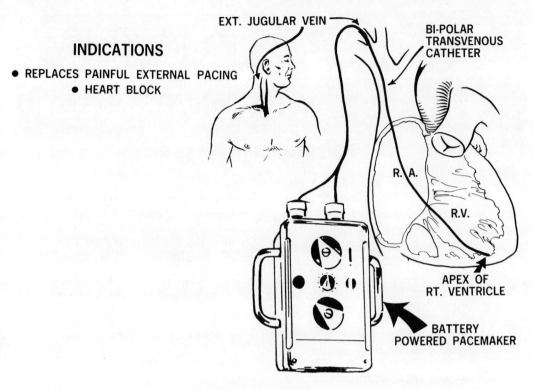

INDICATIONS

- REPLACES PAINFUL EXTERNAL PACING
  - HEART BLOCK

EXT. JUGULAR VEIN

BI-POLAR
TRANSVENOUS
CATHETER

R. A.

R.V.

APEX OF
RT. VENTRICLE

BATTERY
POWERED PACEMAKER

FIG. 12–1. Endocardial pacing.

of the right ventricle using fluoroscopic control. The proximal end of the electrode catheter is then attached to a small demand or stand-by battery-powered pacemaker. Figure 12–1 shows a battery-operated pacemaker attached to a bipolar transvenous catheter positioned in the apex of the right ventricle.

The demand pacemaker detects the ventricular R wave, and electrical stimulation takes place only if ventricular contraction fails to occur within the preset time interval.

Two settings are made on the pacemaker:

1. The output control, which adjusts the amplitude of the pacing impulses from 0.5 to 25 milliamperes.
2. The rate control, which is usually set to deliver from 60 to 75 impulses per minute.

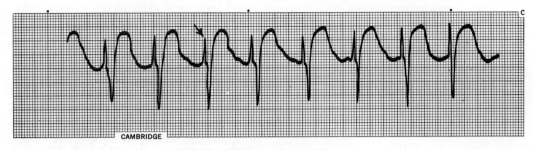

Fig. 12–2. Artificial pacemaker spike.

Figure 12–2 presents an artificial pacemaker spike. The above strip was taken on an 84-year-old man, with a transvenous pacemaker in place, for second degree heart block with Wenckebach, and alternating left and right bundle branch block, following an acute myocardial infarction. The pacemaker is rate-fixed at 82, is firing regularly and having a 1:1 response.

Figure 12–3 presents pacemaker electrode displacement. The strip shows failure of electronic pacemaker stimuli to capture in a transvenous catheter pacemaker.

Figure 12–4 is the same pacemaker after repositioning of the catheter electrode, showing 1:1 capture.

NURSING RESPONSIBILITIES

1. Watch for infection.
2. Note any symptoms of thrombus formation.
3. Be sure electrode and circuitry are checked.
4. Be sure batteries are tested periodically.
5. Monitor and synchronize atrial/radial pulse and oscilloscope.

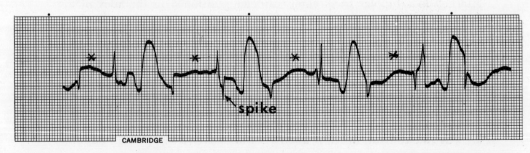

Fig. 12–3. Pacemaker electrode displacement. The asterisks represent noncapture.

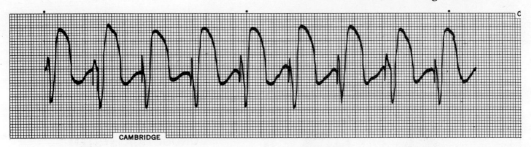

CAMBRIDGE

FIG. 12–4. Catheter repositioned.

The catheter is sutured in place at the point of insertion. Sterile cleansing of this area is necessary to prevent infection. A break in sterile technique while inserting the catheter may result in phlebitis.

Injury to the lining of the vein used to insert the catheter may cause thrombosis. Occasionally, in the process of removing the temporary transvenous pacing catheter, the radial pulse of the arm used is abolished by accidental ligation of the vessel. This is a benign phenomenon which requires no treatment since collateral circulation develops rapidly.

Frequent battery and electrode tests are necessary to determine if the pacemaker is functioning properly. The checking procedure depends upon the pacemaker model. Testing for a broken or shortened electrode is necessary. The number of hours the batteries are used should be accurately recorded. Their voltage output should be regularly checked in order to insure proper amplitude.

The patient on a pacemaker is monitored for at least three days. Close observation of the ECG is important to determine pacemaker function and to note any rhythm disturbances.

The pacemaker impulse produces a pacing artifact, indicated by a sharp downward or upward deflection preceding each QRS complex.

If the patient is not monitored, the apical pulse is taken to check the heart rate and rhythm. The radial pulse is taken to determine if the beats are strong enough to maintain circulation.

PERMANENT CARDIAC PACING

Prior to the development of electronic pacemakers, the person with heart block or a low cardiac output, as in Adams-Stokes syndrome, had a poor prognosis. With artificial pacing, many have been restored to an active life.

There are two approaches to pacemaker implantations:

1. Permanent pacing may be accomplished by use of a transvenous endocardial catheter with a pacemaker impulse generator implanted sub-

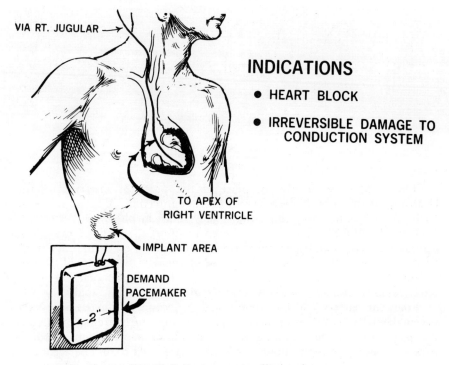

VIA RT. JUGULAR →

INDICATIONS

● HEART BLOCK

● IRREVERSIBLE DAMAGE TO
   CONDUCTION SYSTEM

TO APEX OF
RIGHT VENTRICLE

IMPLANT AREA

DEMAND
PACEMAKER

2"

FIG. 12–5. Permanent cardiac pacing.

cutaneously in the pectoralis muscle. This approach is shown in Figure 12–5.
2. The transthoracic approach is accomplished by implanting the electrodes directly on the myocardium and connecting them to a pulse generator implanted subcutaneously in the abdominal wall.

Indications for permanent pacing are:

1. Heart block
2. Irreversible damage to the conduction system

Permanent heart block is associated with a variety of conditions, including atherosclerosis, valvular disease, surgical trauma and acute infectious diseases.

Changes in the conduction system may result from disease processes such as syphilis, myocarditis or endocarditis. Congenital heart block is rare, but may be associated with congenital heart defects such as tetralogy of Fallot or a ventricular septal defect.

Symptoms of heart block vary from none to the disabling Adams-Stokes attack. Diagnostic studies include laboratory tests, chest x-rays and

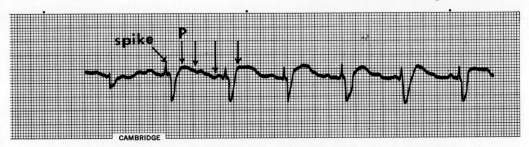

Fɪɢ. 12–6. Atrial tachycardia with third-degree A-V block.

an ECG. Diagnosis is confirmed by the ECG, which shows a complete dissociation between the atrial and ventricular rhythms, with a slow ventricular rate. Surgical implantation of an electric pacemaker is indicated if medical treatment is inadequate.

NURSING RESPONSIBILITIES

Preoperative

1. Prepare for diagnostic studies.
2. Assist the patient in accepting the pacemaker. The patient will undoubtedly experience apprehension and anxiety. Emotional support must include an explanation of why the implant is being done as well as a simple explanation of the procedure and the postoperative program.
3. Preoperative teaching should also include teaching the patient to cough and breathe deeply.

Postoperative

1. Control pain.
2. Monitor.
3. Evaluate effectiveness of the pacemaker.
4. Check vital signs.
5. Teach patient how to deep breathe and cough.

Use of the transthoracic approach to implant the pacemaker causes considerable pain. Narcotic analgesics should be given as ordered to keep the patient comfortable and to relieve his anxiety.

Monitoring is necessary to evaluate the effectiveness of the pacemaker. The apical beat, radial pulse and oscilloscope must synchronize.

Vital signs should be checked for rate and rhythm disturbances.

Coughing and deep breathing should be carried out at least every two hours to increase pulmonary volume.

Figure 12–6 presents atrial tachycardia with third-degree A-V block, with an implanted pacemaker. In this ECG strip, atrial P waves of changing contour fall at a rate of 240 plus. The artificial pacemaker is firing at 70 times per minute, with 1:1 response.

Types of Permanent Pacemakers

1. The **fixed-rate pacemaker,** which sends an impulse through the electrode at a rate set between 60 to 75 impulses per minute; it completely controls the pacing of the heart.
2. The **synchronized pacemaker,** which sends atrial impulses to the pulse generator, which then stimulates the ventricles; it is usually set so that the ventricles beat in response to atrial contractions. The synchronized pacemaker has built-in safety features, such as a mechanism to prevent tachycardias. If the atrial rate exceeds 110, the pacer blocks alternate beats, thus setting up a 2:1 block.
3. The **demand pacemaker,** which is designed to function when the heart rate drops below the prefixed level; each QRS complex is sensed and programs a timing device in the pacemaker; stimulation occurs when the normal heart rate is lower than the pacemaker rate.

The nursing care should include teaching the patient and his family how to check his pulse morning and evening. The patient should notify his physician if there is any variation in the pulse rate or if he experiences any dizziness or syncope.

The batteries in the pacemaker are designed to last five years. Most physicians recommend that they be replaced every two or three years.

ELECTRICAL SAFETY FACTORS

The maintenance of electrical safety in hospitals has always been a major concern of hospital administrators and engineers, especially in regard to operating room areas because of the presence of explosive gases. All electrically operated devices have the potential for voltage leakage. In most cases, where this leakage does not exceed certain limits, this hazard is well taken care of by proper grounding, which carries the leaking current through a wire to a distant ground point, where it poses no electrical hazard to the user of the instrument.

Prevention consists of maintaining electrical standards for equipment, such as wall plugs and sockets, and wiring down to ground point. The third prong on the wall plug leads to ground point when inserted into an electrical outlet designed to carry stray current to earth.

Many articles are still brought into hospitals with no arrangement for grounding to built-in ground. These include portable plug-in radios, heating pads, portable plug-in television sets and hair dryers. The omission of grounding is evident in the presence of a two-pronged plug, rather than a three-pronged plug.

With the proliferation of electrically operated monitoring equipment, a new element of hazard has been introduced, in that the devices are attached to the patient and the patient thus becomes a part of the electrical circuit. The problem is compounded when more than one such apparatus is attached to a patient; for example, a cardiac monitor plus one or more ECG machines, portable suction pump, hypothermia blankets, vaporizers, electrical beds, and so on.

If one or more of these devices were to have a current leakage which exceeds the threshold of resistance of the patient's intact skin, then such leakage runs off to ground through a circuit that includes the patient's body. Such leakage current is increased whenever more than one instrument is plugged into the same power source.

The ECG machine, with its multiple attachments to the patient, enhances the possibility of accidental shock to the patient. Thus, when an ECG is being taken, the patient should be disconnected from all other electrical devices, including monitors.

It has been found that a current of 116 milliamperes can cause fibrillation of the heart, if it crosses the patient's chest, arm to arm. Where needle electrodes are used, the protective intact skin threshold is reduced considerably, and much less current is required to produce fibrillation.

If accidental current is introduced to a transvenous catheter in the patient's atrium, the threshold for fibrillation is reduced to 20–35 milliamperes. This amount of current applied to the intact skin is imperceptible to the senses. The intact skin threshold for perceptible shock is approximately 1000 microamperes.

Leakage current can be introduced through the pacemaker catheter if poor protection exists at the electrode attachment to the pacemaker pack. If a nurse or doctor touches the controls of the pacemaker pack and simultaneously touches other equipment with leakage voltage, such as an electrical bed or an ECG machine, this current may then be delivered to the heart. If the person touching the controls of the pacemaker pack wears dry rubber gloves, this transfer of current cannot occur. It is suggested that the entire pacemaker pack be encased in a transparent rubber glove, and that controls be operated through the rubber glove at all times.

To contribute to the electrical safety of the patient in the coronary care unit:

1. The electrical engineer should regularly check wall outlets for proper grounding.
2. Check for leakage voltage. Instruments are available for checking leakage voltage when several electrical devices are used simultaneously. Such checking should be done under operating conditions. Maximum allowable leakage is probably 5 microamperes.

3. Never use "cheaters" to plug two-pronged plugs into three-pronged outlets. No grounding exists when the "pig-tail" has not been properly attached to the wall outlet plate.

4. Never use a three-pronged plug that has been damaged. Chances are that the grounding wire has been broken.

5. Check equipment daily; if wires are broken or frayed, have the equipment repaired before using.

6. Never use needle electrodes when the patient is attached to another electrically operated device such as an ECG machine.

7. Do not use or permit the patient to touch any equipment that does not have a three-pronged plug.

REFERENCES AND BIBLIOGRAPHY

Arnow, S., Bruner, J. M. R., Siegal, E. F., and Sloss, L. J.: Ventricular fibrillation associated with an electrically operated bed. New Eng. J. Med. *281*:1, (July) 1969.

Briller, S. A.: Electrocution hazards. *In* Driefus, L. S., and Likoff, W.: Mechanism and Therapy of Cardiac Arrhythmias. New York, Grune and Stratton, 1966.

Bruner, J. M. R.: Hazards of electrical apparatus, Anesthesiology, *28*:396, 1967.

Burchell, H., and Strum, R. E.: Electroshock hazards. Circulation, *35*:227, 1967.

Cross, E., Paper presented at Michigan Heart Association Regional Seminar on Intensive Coronary Care, Flint, Michigan, May 25, 1966.

Friedberg, C. K.: Diseases of the Heart. ed. 3. pp. 219-242, 284-304, 443-474, 483-575, 583-628, 643-693, 676-678, 706-791, 866-922. Philadelphia, W. B. Saunders, 1966.

Hospitals: Too many shocks. Time, pp. 58, 63, April 18, 1969.

Medical World News. pp. 30-31, August 23, 1968.

Meltzer, L. E.: *et al.:* Intensive Coronary Care—A Manual for Nurses. CCU Fund, Philadelphia Presbyterian Hospital, 1965.

Merkel, R., and Sovie, M.: Electrocution hazards with transvenous pacemaker electrodes. Am. J. Nurs. *68*:2560-2564, (Dec.) 1968.

Proceedings of the National Conference on Coronary Care Units. p. 25. Washington, D.C., U.S. Dept. of Health, Education and Welfare, 1968.

Whalen, R. E., and Starmer, C. F.: Electrical shock hazards in clinical cardiology. Mod. Conc. Cardio. Dis., *32*:7, 1967.

13 ACTIONS OF DRUGS COMMONLY USED IN CARDIAC CARE

The administration of medications is an important nursing responsibility. There is no room for error since there are no harmless drugs. The nurse should be familiar with any drug she gives since any medication that is capable of helping a patient is also capable of injuring him.

DIGITALIS

Digitalis encompasses a group of naturally-occurring glycosides and their refinements which simultaneously exert beneficial as well as toxic effects on the heart. They differ from each other in potency, time of onset and duration of effect.

EFFECT ON NORMAL HEART

One most important effect of digitalis is to increase the contractile force of heart muscle, resulting in increased cardiac output. Theoretically, digitalis influences the diffusion of calcium, potassium and sodium across the cell membrane. Calcium acts as a catalyst in producing muscle contractions.

Conductivity, refractoriness and automaticity are all influenced by digitalis, but the drug has different qualitative and quantitative effects in different areas of the heart.

1. In the S-A node, the automaticity is decreased.
2. In the atria, conduction is slowed, refractoriness is prolonged and automaticity is increased.
3. In the A-V node, conduction is slowed, refractoriness is prolonged and automaticity is increased.
4. In the Purkinje tissue, conduction is accelerated, refractoriness is decreased and automaticity is increased.
5. In the ventricles, automaticity is increased.

171

ECG changes occur because of an alteration of the repolarization process in the presence of digitalis. Normally the ventricular walls are repolarized from the epicardial to the endocardial surface. After digitalis, however, repolarization of the ventricular wall occurs sooner, due to more rapid conduction, decreased refractoriness, increased automaticity and deviation of the repolarization process from the normal pathway. If recovery begins before excitation is completed, the two processes overlap. All this appears in the ECG as a shortened Q-T interval, a sagging S-T, and a depressed or inverted T wave.

These are essentially the early changes which occur in myocardial infarction. When digitalis is used in the presence of myocardial infarction, it is not always possible to determine positively which ECG effects are due to the drug and which to the disease.

The systemic action of digitalis results in:

1. An increased cardiac output
2. A stabilized fluid balance by improved renal function
3. Mobilization of the fluid of edema of cardiac failure
4. Reduced right atrial pressure

TOXICITY

ECG changes resulting from digitalis therapy include:

1. Sinus bradycardia
2. P-R prolongation
3. A-V dissociation
4. Ventricular arrhythmias
5. Atrial arrhythmias, with some degree of block

Systemic changes resulting from digitalis therapy include:

1. Anorexia, nausea, diarrhea and vomiting
2. Yellow or green vision, referred to as "halo" vision
3. Drowsiness, headache and confusion

USES

1. Heart failure
2. Atrial fibrillation
3. Atrial flutter
4. Supraventricular tachycardia

DOSAGE

A heart is said to be *digitalized* when its cells have been saturated to the therapeutic point and before the point of toxicity. The amount of drug necessary to achieve this effect is determined by the pretreatment condition of the heart in all of its properties. In other words, the *digitalizing dose* for any patient is that dose which will produce the desired effect in *that* patient. The *maintenance dose* is that dose which will maintain therapeutic saturation, and is governed by the rate at which the patient metabolizes and excretes the drug.

The physician may elect to achieve a saturation point in varying periods of time, according to the urgency of the patient's condition, such as:

1. Very rapid digitalization—12 hours or less
2. Rapid digitalization—12 to 24 hours
3. Moderate digitalization—2 days
4. Slow digitalization—3 to 7 days

Regardless of the digitalis preparation used or the route of administration, the physician will probably use standardized dosages as a departure-point for individualizing the dosage.

TABLE 13–1. DIGITALIS PREPARATIONS

DRUG	MODE	DURATION OF EFFECT	AVERAGE DIGITALIZATION DOSE	MAINTENANCE DOSE
Ouabain	I.V.	24–48 hrs.	0.8–1.0 mg.	
Cedilanid	I.V.	36–72 hrs.	1.6 mg.	
Digoxin	I.V. oral	24–48 hrs.	3–4 mg.	0.25–0.75 mg.
Gitalin	I.V. oral	24–72 hrs.	5–7 mg.	0.25–1.0 mg.
Digitoxin	I.V. oral	1–3 weeks	1.2–2 mg.	0.1–2 mg.
Digitalis leaf	Oral	2–3 weeks	1.02–2 Gm.	0.1–0.15 Gm.

CONTRAINDICATIONS
1. Idiosyncracy
2. Digitalis intoxication
3. High-degree A-V block

CAUTIONS
1. Digitalization in myocardial infarction should be accomplished slowly because of myocardial irritability.
2. Digitalis should be given I.V. or I.M. only in acute pulmonary edema or other life-threatening situations. If there is doubt concerning previous digitalis therapy, small doses should be used and repeated to obtain the desired effect.

3. Potassium depletion from diuretics may precipitate toxicity.
4. Sudden deaths have occurred on administering intravenous calcium to digitalized patients.
5. Tolerance and dose-requirement may be reduced in concomitant disease such as debilitated old age, myxedema, myocarditis, myocardial infarction, renal insufficiency, electrolyte disturbance and advanced pulmonary disease.
6. Predisposition to arrhythmia may occur with concurrent drug administration, such as ephedrine, epinephrine, reserpine, procainamide or quinidine.

QUINIDINE

Quinidine and quinine alkaloids are derived from the cinchona bark. Quinidine is chemically the same as quinine, but with a different molecular structure.

PHARMACOLOGICAL EFFECTS

1. Rhythm function is depressed and ectopic pacemakers are more depressed than the S-A node.
2. Depolarization rate is decreased.
3. Intraventricular and A-V conduction velocity is slowed and conduction time is prolonged.
4. Intracardiac vagal block occurs. The A-V refractory period is shortened, allowing passage of more impulses from the atria when the atria are beating or fibrillating at a rapid rate. Digitalis is usually given prior to the use of quinidine in order to defeat this mechanism and to slow the rate of ventricular response.[1]
5. Myocardial contractility is depressed.
6. There is a peripheral adrenergic blockade which produces vasodilation and hypotension.
7. Quinidine can produce ectopic ventricular tachycardia.

ECG FINDINGS

1. Prolongation of the P-R interval
2. Prolongation of the QRS interval
3. Prolongation of the Q-T segment
4. Flattened or inverted T wave
5. Tall U waves

---

[1] Smith, J. W.: Manual of Medical Therapeutics. ed. 19, p. 118. Boston, Little, Brown and Co., 1969.

LABORATORY TEST FINDINGS
1. Increased prothrombin time
2. Increased urine catecholamines
3. Direct positive influence on Coombs test[2]

TOXIC EFFECTS
1. **In the absence of arrhythmia:** nausea, vomiting, abdominal cramps, diarrhea, tinnitus, double vision, light-headedness, premature ventricular beats, ventricular tachycardia or fibrillation, hypotension and prolongation of the QRS interval by more than 25 per cent, or greater than 0.14 second. A 50 per cent widening of the QRS interval may produce ventricular fibrillation.
2. **In the presence of arrhythmia:** atrial flutter with rapid ventricular response, A-V dissociation, asystole (due to depression of atrial pacemaker), with or without syncope or convulsion.

ALLERGIC REACTIONS
1. Fever
2. Asthma
3. Urticaria
4. Purpura

It is recommended that whenever possible, a test dose be given to rule out allergy.

CONTRAINDICATIONS
1. Atrial arrhythmia with A-V block, whether produced by digitalis or a disease process
2. Bundle branch block or intraventricular block
3. Acute rheumatic fever or bacterial endocarditis
4. Third trimester of pregnancy
5. Untreated thyrotoxicosis
6. Congestive heart failure

USES
1. Paroxysmal supraventricular arrhythmias
2. Digitalis toxicity with atrial or nodal tachycardia and frequent premature ventricular beats
3. Premature ventricular beats
4. Recurrent ventricular tachycardia
5. The Wolff-Parkinson-White accelerated conduction syndrome

---

2 Meyers, F. H., Jawetz, E., and Goldfien, E.: Review of Medical Pharmacology. p. 660. Los Altos, California, Lange Medical Publications, 1968.

DOSAGE

Regardless of the route of administration, the aim is to reach and maintain therapeutic serum drug levels. When feasible, dosage should be adjusted to periodic serum level determinations:

1. **Oral or intramuscular:** 0.2 Gm. every 6 hours around the clock, regulating dosage to response.
2. **Intravenous:** 0.8 Gm. in 100 cc. of 5% glucose in distilled water, titrated to administer 1.0 ml. per minute, or 300-500 mg. over a 30–60 minute period.

Sustained release preparations of quinidine are available, but have not yet received general acceptance. The severe cardio-toxic effects of quinidine are treated with intravenous molar lactate.

CAUTIONS

1. The ECG should be monitored frequently for QRS interval widening.
2. The drug should be stopped if the QRS interval widens by 50 per cent.
3. In the presence of bundle branch block, the drug should be stopped if the QRS interval widens by 25 per cent.
4. The drug should be discontinued if severe vomiting or frequent premature ventricular beats occur.

PROCAINAMIDE (PRONESTYL)

Procainamide hydrochloride is a chemically altered procaine, which is a local anesthetic. It is more stable than procaine.

It is believed that one effect of local anesthetics is the prevention of an increased permeability of cell membrane to sodium, which is the first step in depolarization.

ACTION

With systemic absorption of local anesthetics, central nervous system stimulation can occur, sometimes followed by depression. Stimulation of respiratory, vasomotor, and vagal centers may produce increased respiratory minute volume, rise in blood pressure, bradycardia, vomiting and convulsions.

Procainamide has the same antiarrhythmic effect as quinidine. However, quinidine is more likely to depress the atrial pacemakers, while procainamide is more likely to produce premature beats or tachycardia.

The systemic toxic effects are the same as quinidine, minus the classical symptoms of cinchonism (salivation, tinnitus, headache, dizziness, visual disturbances and confusion).

A Lupus-like syndrome has occasionally been seen as a symptom of procainamide toxicity.

CONTRAINDICATIONS

1. A-V block
2. Sensitivity manifested by hives, chills, fever, angioedema

USES

1. It is sometimes used to replace quinidine in quinidine-sensitive patients.
2. Premature ventricular beats
3. Ventricular tachycardia
4. Premature ventricular beats of digitalis toxicity
5. Premature atrial beats, especially if frequent or multifocal
6. Prior to elective cardioversion

DOSAGE

For premature ventricular beats, 250 to 500 mg. are given orally every 6 hours.

For ventricular tachycardia, it should be diluted and given no more rapidly than 50 mg. per minute, intravenously. Because of its tendency to produce hypotension, blood pressure should be monitored every 2 minutes during intravenous administration, and the ECG should be monitored continuously for signs of cardio-toxicity (excessive QRS interval widening and drug-induced arrhythmia).

Note: The severe cardio-toxic effects of procainamide are usually treated by withdrawal of the drug and administration of I.V. molar lactate.

LIDOCAINE

Lidocaine (Xylocaine) is a local anesthetic agent currently used intravenously for its antiarrhythmic properties. It was first used for this purpose by Hitchcock and Keown in 1958 in the treatment of bigeminy incidental to cardiac surgery.

It acts at the cell-membrane level by influencing permeability to sodium, potassium and other ions. As a consequence, generation and conduction of the impulse are inhibited. There is little depression of the S-A node.

Its actions are essentially those of procainamide, but dose for dose, it is more potent. It has a rapid onset of action due to its diffusibility. It is thought to be superior to procainamide because it decreases ventricular excitability without depressing contractile force, and is not as prone to produce hypotension.

USES

1. As a supplement to general anesthesia for its antiarrhythmic effect
2. To facilitate electrical defibrillation

3. To terminate ventricular arrhythmias incidental to cardiac catheterization
4. As a substitute for quinidine or procainamide in patients who have had allergic reactions to these drugs
5. For digitalis-induced premature ventricular beats
6. For ventricular tachycardia when electrical cardioversion is not indicated, advisable or available

CONTRAINDICATIONS

1. Liver disorders (Lidocaine is metabolized in the liver.)
2. A-V dissociation with a slow nodal or ventricular pacemaker. Further slowing due to the drug may produce increased ectopic ventricular activity.

TOXIC EFFECTS

1. Analgesia and drowsiness
2. Difficulty in breathing or swallowing
3. Blurring of vision or double vision
4. Numbness
5. Sweating
6. Cerebral irritation—coma, convulsion and respiratory arrest

DOSAGE

1. 50–100 mg. as the initial dose
2. Intravenous drip of 1.0–2 mg. per minute

To prepare intravenous infusion:

1. *Objective:* to deliver 2 mg. lidocaine per minute
   a. Use 500 cc. bottle of 5% in D/W.
   b. Discard 100 cc.
   c. Add to bottle 100 cc. of 1% lidocaine solution (10 mg./cc.), giving a total of 1000 mg. of drug.
   d. The prepared solution now contains 2 mg. per cc.
   e. Use microdrip at a rate of 60 per minute.
2. *Objective:* to deliver 1.0 mg. lidocaine per minute.
   Use above solution at a rate of 30 microdrops per minute.
3. *Objective:* to deliver 0.5 mg. of lidocaine per minute.
   Use above solution at a rate of 15 microdrops per minute.

Caution: A preparation of lidocaine mixed with epinephrine is available for local anesthesia. It carries a red label. It should *never* be substituted for plain lidocaine. As a safety factor, in order to avoid accidental substitution, the red-labeled lidocaine should never be stocked in the coronary care unit.

DILANTIN (DIPHENYLHYDANTOIN)

Dilantin is a drug chemically related to the barbiturates, long used for its antiseizure effect in epilepsy without causing sedation.

It prevents the spread of abnormal electrical activity by counteracting excess sodium leakage into the cell. It is now being used experimentally in the treatment of cardiac arrhythmias.

USES

Dilantin is used in the treatment of premature ventricular beats and ventricular tachycardia, especially if induced by digitalis. It is believed that it counteracts the ectopic effects of digitalis without altering its inotropic effect.

TOXIC EFFECT

1. Toxic effects of long-term therapy, as in the treatment of epilepsy, are not relevant here.
2. Toxic effects of short-term intensive use:
   a. Ataxia, drowsiness, confusion, nystagmus, tremors
   b. Sinus bradycardia and A-V conduction disturbances
   c. Ventricular fibrillation and asystole have occurred in elderly, debilitated patients.

DOSAGE

1. **Oral:** 100 to 200 mg. t.i.d.
2. **Intramuscular:** 100 mg.
3. **Intravenous:** 125 mg. diluted to 25 mg. per cc. over a 5-minute period. May be given as quickly as 500 mg. per hour. Dose should not exceed 1.0 Gm. per day.

Note: Dilantin may color the urine red to red-brown. It may enhance the effect of coumarin drugs. There is a low tolerance for the drug in liver disease. It is not recommended for use in hypoxia or acidosis.

PROPRANOLOL (INDERAL)

Propranolol is a beta-adrenergic blocking agent which blocks the cardiac and vasodilating effects of epinephrine and the cardiac effects of norepinephrine. It is more effective in ventricular than atrial arrhythmias.

CARDIAC EFFECTS
1. Decrease in normal sinus rate and atrial pacemaker rate
2. Slowed A-V conduction
3. Reduced force of contraction
4. Quinidine-like effect on ectopic foci

USES
1. **Atrial flutter or fibrillation:** reduces ventricular rate due to slowed A-V conduction. Slows atrial ectopic rates. (Digitalis is still the drug of choice.)
2. **Digitalis-induced arrhythmia:** atrial tachycardia, ventricular tachycardia, multiple premature ventricular beats
3. **Ventricular tachycardia** if cardioversion is not available
4. **Prevention of anginal pain** due to reduction of cardiac work

SIDE EFFECTS
Dizziness, tiredness, depression, gastro-intestinal disturbances, paresthesias, muscle aching and asthma

TOXIC EFFECTS
1. **Oral:** congestive failure, hypotension, A-V block, laryngospasm, bronchiolar constriction
2. **I. V.:** bradycardia, A-V block with very slow idioventricular rate
3. **Reactions:** rash and thrombocytopenic purpura

CONTRAINDICATIONS
1. Congestive failure
2. Hypotension
3. Complete heart block
4. Asthma or other pulmonary disease
5. Not to be given concurrently with:
   a. Eutonyl
   b. Parnate
   c. Reserpine
   d. Guanethidine
   e. Methyldopa

DOSAGE
1. **Oral:** 10 to 40 mg. t.i.d.
2. **I. V.:** 1.03 to 3 mg., slower than 1.0 mg. per minute, with the patient being monitored continuously

Table 13–2 presents a list of drugs and treatments according to preferred usage in treating the more common arrhythmias.

TABLE 13–2. THERAPY IN ARRHYTHMIA IN ORDER OF PROBABLE CHOICE*

	DIGITALIS	QUINIDINE	INDEROL	LIDOCAINE	DILANTIN	PRONESTYL	OTHER
1. Atrial flutter or fibrillation	1						2 Cardioversion†
2. Uncontrolled atrial flutter or fibrillation			2				1 Cardioversion†
3. Regular supraventricular tachycardia	2		4		3		1 Vasopressors / 2 Cardioversion†
4. Recurrent supraventricular tachycardia		1	3		2	1	
5. Ventricular tachycardia		4	5	1	2	4	3 Cardioversion†
6. Recurrent ventricular tachycardia		1	3		2	1	
7. Premature ventricular beats		1	3		2	1	
8. Premature ventricular beats and heart failure	1	2			3	2	
9. Ventricular fibrillation				1			Defibrillation
10. Post-defibrillation for ventricular fibrillation		1	4	3	2	1	
11. Digitalis toxicity with:							
a. Atrial tachycardia, with or without block		3	1		2	3	Plus potassium
b. Nodal tachycardia		3	1		2	3	Plus potassium
c. Many premature supraventricular beats		3	1		2	3	Plus potassium
d. Premature ventricular beats		1	2		3	1	Plus potassium
e. Ventricular tachycardia with heart failure		3	4	1	2	3	Plus potassium

* Numbers 1–5 indicated order of choice.
† Cardioversion should always be preceded and followed by Pronestyl or quinidine.

ATROPINE

Atropine is a naturally occurring alkaloid of atropa belladonna. Its action is parasympatholytic by blocking the effect of acetylcholine.

EFFECTS

In small doses, the pulse may slow. In larger doses, the vagus influence is blocked and pulse rate speeds up. The blood pressure in the recumbent position may be slightly elevated. Postural hypotension may occur in the erect position after an injected dose. The T wave may be lowered in the ECG.

USES

1. To abolish vagus influence in syncope due to S-A block
2. For ventricular tachycardia, to abolish vagus influence and lengthen refractory period of ventricular muscle
3. For heart block due to vagotonia
4. For heart block with slow ventricular rate, to stimulate an increase in ventricular rate
5. To lessen the degree of partial heart block, by abolishing vagus influence on the A-V node

CONTRAINDICATIONS

Glaucoma, gastric dilatation or retention, and urinary retention

TOXIC EFFECTS

1. Classic systemic atropine effects
2. A-V block and nodal rhythm

DOSAGE

In sinus bradycardia or second-degree A-V block—0.3 to 1.2 mg. I.V. every 4 hours

Adams-Stokes attacks—0.5 to 1.0 mg. (H) t.i.d. or q.i.d.

VASOCONSTRICTORS AND VASODILATORS

The vasopressor drugs play a large role in the treatment of shock, regardless of its cause. The therapeutic aim is the restoration of normal blood flow to vital areas. Normal blood pressure usually means adequate tissue perfusion. However, because blood pressure is a summation of peripheral resistance, cardiac output and cardiac rate, this is not necessarily so. The normal blood-pressure reading may have been obtained at the expense of traumatic vasoconstriction in some vital zone. Much interest is presently being shown in the role of vasodilation in the treatment of shock.

The mechanism of shock is not clearly understood. Therefore, treatment of shock is based on clinical experience. Most clinical experience has been in the use of vasoconstricting drugs. Whether the physician chooses a vasoconstrictor or a vasodilator in any particular instance, the underlying principle of the treatment is the antagonism or the augmentation of physiological responses.

In order to understand the effects of the vasoconstrictor and vasodilator drugs, it is necessary to review briefly the effects of the sympathetic and the parasympathetic nervous system.

Sympathetic and parasympathetic nervous system stimulation sometimes causes stimulating and sometimes inhibiting effects in specific organs. Ususally, if sympathetic stimulation causes stimulating effects, parasympathetic stimulation acts as an antagonist and is inhibitory. Most often, the individual organ is dominated by one or the other system.

Here we are concerned with the major effects of the nervous system upon the cardiovascular system.

Parasympathetic Mechanism

1. Acetylcholine is stored at parasympathetic nerve endings. These fibers, which secrete acetylcholine, are said to be cholinergic.
2. Parasympathetic stimulation triggers release of acetylcholine at nerve endings. On release, acetylcholine stimulates muscle fibers.
3. Immediately after release of acetylcholine, cholinesterase, an enzyme which inactivates or destroys acetylcholine, is released.
4. In heart muscle, acetylcholine is an inhibitory transmitter, because it increases cell-membrane permeability to potassium, thus rendering heart muscle less excitable and slowing heart rate.
5. Drugs which affect neuromuscular junction:
   a. *Nicotine-like,* which affect transmission of the impulse by acetylcholine-like action
   b. *Curare-like,* which block transmission of the impulse by antagonizing the effect of acetylcholine
   c. *Neostigmine-like,* which stimulate the transmission of the impulse at the neural junction by inactivating cholinesterase

Sympathetic Mechanism

1. Norepinephrine and small amounts of epinephrine are stored at sympathetic nerve endings. Those fibers which secrete these chemicals are said to be adrenergic.
2. Sympathetic nervous stimulation triggers the release of norepinephrine and epinephrine at the nerve endings.
3. In cardiac muscle, norepinephrine is an excitatory transmitter inasmuch as it increases cell-membrane permeability to all ions.

Adrenal Medullary Mechanism

1. In the adrenal medulla, sympathetic nervous stimulation triggers the release of norepinephrine and epinephrine into the blood stream.
2. When these blood-borne chemicals reach the effectors of an organ, they have the same effect as the chemicals usually stored at the nerve endings, but have an action of longer duration. They can act as a supplement to or a substitute for the central nervous system effect.
3. In addition, the blood-borne secretions of the adrenal medulla can stimulate body structures not directly supplied with nerve fibers from the central nervous system.

Alpha and Beta Mechanism

Epinephrine and norepinephrine produce distinct yet overlapping responses at the neural junction. To explain this, it has been postulated that two types of substances must exist in the effector cell:

1. **Alpha receptor substance:** affected by norepinephrine. Activation of alpha receptors results in vasoconstriction in the skin, splanchnic area and muscle.
2. **Beta receptor substance:** affected by both norepinephrine and epinephrine. Activation of beta receptors results in vasodilation, increased cardiac rate and force of cardiac contraction.

Adrenergic Drugs

The adrenergic drugs (sympathomimetic) are those which imitate in whole or in part the effects of sympathetic nerve stimulation or adrenal medullary discharge.

1. **Catecholamines** (epinephrine, norepinephrine, isoproterenol), which act directly on effector cells.
2. **Ephedrine and ephedrine variants,** which act indirectly through body catecholamines.

Adrenergic Blocking Drugs

Adrenergic blocking agents are a part of that group of drugs (sympathoplegic) which block the action of sympathomimetic amines or limit sympathetic outflow.

1. **Alpha-adrenergic:** act on the effector organ to antagonize the vasoconstricting effects of epinephrine and norepinephrine: for example, Regitine and Dibenzyline.
2. **Beta-adrenergic:** act on the effector organ to antagonize the cardiac effects and vasodilating effects of epinephrine, and the cardiac effects of norepinephrine; for example, propranalol.

DRUGS COMMONLY USED IN RESUSCITATION

1. Sodium bicarbonate, I.V., to combat acidosis:
   a. 500 cc. of 5% sodium bicarbonate, containing 298 mEq., at a rate of 80-100 cc. per minute (Calcium solutions must not be given through the same tubing.)
   b. Direct injection into vein, 50-cc. amp. of 7.5% solution, containing 45 mEq., every 5 to 10 minutes until cardiac activity is restored
2. Calcium chloride, I.V. or intracardiac, to strengthen force of cardiac contraction: give 10 cc. of 10% solution. Not to be used if patient is digitalized. Especially indicated for patients in hyperkalemia or hypocalcemia.
3. Hydrocortisone, 300 mg. I.V. for adrenal insufficiency
4. Dibenzyline Phenoxybenzamine, alpha-adrenergic blocking agent, to counteract inappropriate and prolonged peripheral vasoconstriction: one mg. per kg. I.V. Should not be used in heart failure.
5. Dextran, to expand blood volume: give 500 cc. by I.V. drip, measuring central venous pressure.
6. Potassium chloride, to convert arrhythmias due to digitalis: give 40 mEq. in 500 cc. 5% in D/W over a 2- to 3-hour period.
   a. If the serum potassium level is above 2.5, no more than 10 mEq. per hour or 200 mEq. per day should be given.
   b. If the serum potassium level is less than 2.0 and electrolyte changes are evident in the ECG, 40 mEq. may be given per hour with no greater concentration than 60 mEq. per liter of I.V., up to 400 mEq. per day.

Table 13–3 presents four vasopressor drugs commonly used in cardiac resuscitation, together with their effects on cardiac output, peripheral resistance and blood pressure, as well as those untoward effects which may occur when they are administered.

TABLE 13–3. EFFECTS OF 4 VASOPRESSOR DRUGS* COMMONLY USED IN CARDIAC RESUSCITATION

DRUG AND DOSE	CARDIAC OUTPUT	PERIPHERAL RESISTANCE	BLOOD PRESSURE	REMARKS
Levarterenol (Levophed): 4–8 mg. in 1000 cc. 5% in D/W by microdrip I.V. infusion, titrated to maintain systolic pressure 30 mm. Hg below patient's normal level	→ or ↕	←	←	May cause slough on infiltration. Regitine may be injected into extravasated site If blood pressure rises too high, may cause reflex bradycardia and lower cardiac output Patient may develop resistance to the drug, requiring an increase in dosage May cause pallor, sweating, vomiting, anxiety, respiratory difficulty, palpitation, headache, photophobia, retro-sternal or pharyngeal pain
Epinephrine (Adrenalin): Dilute 1 cc. of 1:1000 aq. solution in 9 cc. sterile N/S to make 1:10,000. Of this mixture give: I.V., 5 cc. initially Intracardiac, 3 cc. Repeat p.r.n. For continuous I.V. drip use 4 cc. of 1:1,000 in 500 cc. 5% in D/W	←	→	←	May produce ventricular fibrillation or tachycardia in poorly oxygenated heart May produce headache, nervousness, restlessness, pallor, respiratory difficulty, palpitation Sometimes used in heart block to increase nodal and ventricular pacemaker rates

Drug				Remarks
Metaraminol (Aramine): 1 cc. I.M. (10 mg.) if I.V. route not available 0.5 to 5 mg. by I.V. initially 25–100 mg. in 500 cc. 5% in D/W, titrated as for Levophed	←	←	←	Acts by release of norepinephrine, with some direct vasoconstriction May increase cardiac work, slow rate, and lower cardiac output May cause reflex bradycardia Arrhythmia hazard is high Side-effects the same as Levophed
Isoproterenol (Isuprel): 2 mg. in 500 cc. 5% in D/W by microdrip I.V. titrated to ventricular rate of 60–100. Do not use if systolic pressure is less than 80	→	→	←	Less likely to cause ventricular fibrillation than epinephrine Central venous pressure should be monitored May cause tachycardia and ectopic beats May cause skin flushing, sweating, nausea, palpitation, headache, anginal pain, vomiting, nervousness Sometimes used in heart block to increase nodal and ventricular pacemaker rates

* These four drugs increase force of myocardial contraction, heart rate, conductivity of A-V node, and ectopic activity. There is direct stimulation to the S-A node. All are said to increase coronary blood flow.

PROTHROMBIN DEPRESSANTS

Prothrombin depressants inhibit prothrombin synthesis by acting on the synthesis of clotting factors in the liver and thus acting as anticoagulants.

USES

1. For prevention of venous thrombosis in enforced bed rest
2. For acute arterial occlusion
3. For prevention of thrombus formation in atrial fibrillation

AIMS

1. In the first few weeks of therapy, a prothrombin time of 20 to 30 per cent.
2. In maintenance therapy, a prothrombin time of 30 to 40 per cent

COMPLICATIONS OF TREATMENT

1. Hemorrhage occurs in as many as one third of treated patients. Severe hemorrhage occurs in as many as 2 per cent of treated patients.
2. "Rebound" on abrupt cessation of therapy

CONTRAINDICATIONS

1. Bleeding from any site
2. Uncooperative patient
3. Laboratory facilities not available
4. Surgery
5. Hepatic or renal disease
6. Untreated severe hypertension

INCOMPATABILITY

Interaction with other drugs which alter anticoagulant effects; for example, phenobarbital, phenylbutazone, large doses of aspirin

TREATMENT OF OVERDOSE

1. Withdrawal of drug
2. Vitamin K

DOSAGE

All dosages are titrated to responsive changes in prothrombin activity.

1. Dicumarol
   First day—200 to 400 mg.
   Second day—100 to 200 mg.
   Maintenance—25 to 150 mg.

2. Coumadin
   First day—30 to 50 mg.
   Second day—10 to 15 mg.
   Maintenance—5 to 15 mg.
3. Liquamar
   First day—30 mg.
   Second day—10 mg.
   Maintenance—1.0 to 6 mg.
4. Tromexan
   First day—750 to 900 mg. b.i.d.
   Second day—150 to 300 mg. b.i.d.
   Maintenance—150 to 450 mg. b.i.d.
5. Hedulin
   First day—100 to 250 mg. b.i.d.
   Second day—25 to 75 mg. b.i.d.
   Maintenance—12.5 to 75 mg. b.i.d.

HEPARIN

Heparin inhibits thrombin formation and the action of clotting factors in the blood. It is the drug of choice for producing a rapid, anticoagulant effect. It is particularly advantageous because of its rapid absorption and excretion as well as its near nontoxicity. It is almost universally used prior to giving oral anticoagulants.

USES
1. Sudden arterial occlusion
2. Thrombophlebitis

PREPARATION AND DOSAGE
Heparin is supplied in aqueous solution for injection or intravenous use. The strength of the drug is recorded in units per milliliter, and it comes in 1000 to 40,000 units per milliliter preparations. For immediate effect, 3000 to 9000 units I.V. are given every 4 to 6 hours. For prolonged effect 10,000 to 15,000 units are given slowly through a small needle into the subcutaneous fat below the posterior iliac crest. The fat of the abdominal wall may also be used.

The drug may also be given as a continuous intravenous infusion.

The dosage is dependent upon the patient's bleeding and clotting time. The therapeutic level is usually maintained at two to three times the normal clotting time.

CAUTIONS
1. Petechiae in the skin
2. Urinary or rectal bleeding

CONTRAINDICATIONS

1. Bleeding from any site
2. Laboratory facilities not available
3. Hepatic or renal disease
4. Untreated severe hypertension

TREATMENT OF OVERDOSE

1. Withdrawal of drug
2. Whole blood transfusion (fresh blood when possible)
3. Vitamin K
4. Protamine

Table 13–4 presents a list of drugs which may alter the enzyme level as measured by the SGOT and the SGPT. Also listed are drugs which may alter the prothrombin time. It is important that the nurse be aware of such possible effects, since they cause a false diagnosis in the blood study.

TABLE 13–4. SOME DRUGS WHICH MAY ALTER LABORATORY VALUES[1]

SGOT–SGPT	PROTHROMBIN TIME
Acetohexamide (Dymelor)	Aluminum antacids
Allopurinol (Zyloprim)	Aminophylline
Ampicillin	Barbiturates
Bishydroxycoumarin (Dicumarol)	Chloral hydrate
Cephaloridine (Loridine)	Chloramphenicol (Chloromycetin)
Cephalothin (Keflin)	Chlordiazepoxide (Librium)
Chlordiazepoxide (Librium)	Clofibrate (Atromid S)
Clofibrate (Atromid S)	Corticosteroids
Erythromycin	Diphenylhydantoin (Dilantin)
Indomethacin (Indocin)	Ethchlorvynol (Placidyl)
Meperidine (Demerol)	Glutethimide (Doriden)
Methotrexate	Indomethacin (Indocin)
Morphine	Kanamycin
Nalidixic acid (NegGram)	Magnesium antacids
Nitrofurantoin (Fundantin)	Methyldopa (Aldomet)
Oxacillin (Prostaphlin)	Neomycin
Phenacetin	Phenylbutazone (Butazolidin)
Phenothiazine	Quinine
Propranolol (Inderal)	Quinidine
Salicylates	Salicylates
Sulfonamides	Streptomycin
Tetracyclines	Sulfonamides
Tolazamide (Tolinase)	Tetracyclines

[1] Meyers, F. H., Jawetz, E., and Goldfien, A. Review of Medical Pharmacology, pp. 648-662. Los Altos, California, Lange Medical Publications, 1968.

INTRAVENOUS THERAPY

No center in the hospital, except the operating room, has a higher percentage of patients with continuous intravenous infusion than the coronary care unit. This high rate of intravenous therapy is necessary in emergency conditions such as arrhythmia and/or shock which are so frequently encountered by the nurse in the coronary care unit.

The nurse should review her responsibility in this area of patient treatment:

1. Maintain sterile technique whether adding medication to the intravenous solution or giving it through a Y tube.
2. Know the solution. Is it isotonic? The accidental use of saline in a damaged heart can cause cardiac failure.
3. Know the drug and dose to be injected, as well as its normal, untoward toxic and allergic effects. Is the drug fresh? Check the expiration date on the vial. Is the additive drug compatible with the vehicle solution? If more than one drug is added, are they compatible with each other?
   Drugs are incompatible due to:
   a. Chemical effects such as acids and alkalis
   b. Physical effects such as formation of precipitates or other changes in the physical state
   c. Therapeutic incompatibility such as physiological antagonism
   Ask the pharmacist in your hospital for an updated list of drug incompatibilities.
   Drugs susceptible to color changes are packaged in dark bottles to protect them. No drug that has undergone a color change should be used.
4. Some drugs, such as the digitalis preparations, should never be mixed with any other drug or vehicle of administration.

ADVERSE EFFECTS IN INTRAVENOUS THERAPY

1. Idiosyncrasy of dosage—toxic effects of the specific drug.
2. Allergy—anaphylactic shock, urticaria, bronchiospasm, angioedema
3. Pyrogenic, due to introduced organisms—chills, fever, shock
4. Volume overload due to too rapid administration—dyspnea, rales, headache, flushing of skin, nausea, vomiting, irregular pulse
5. Thrombophlebitis—inflammation of a vein near injection site with hardening
6. Extravasation—edema, discoloration at injection site
7. Hematoma—bleeding into tissue at injection site

LEGAL ASPECTS

The nurse must be guided by the nurse-practice laws of her state, the written policy of her hospital and the prevailing custom of peer hospitals of the area in which she practices.

REFERENCES AND BIBLIOGRAPHY

Goodman, L. S., and Gelman, A.: Pharmacological Basis of Therapeutics. ed. 3. New York, Macmillan, 1968.

Guyton, A.: Textbook of Medical Physiology. ed. 3. Philadelphia, W. B. Saunders, 1968.

Hurst, J. W., and Logue, R. R.: The Heart. New York, McGraw-Hill, 1966.

Meyers, R. H., Jawetz, E., and Goldfien, A.: Review of Medical Pharmacology. Los Altos, California, Lange Medical Publications, 1968.

Rodman, M. J., and Smith, D. W.: Pharmacology and Drug Therapy in Nursing. Philadelphia, J. B. Lippincott, 1968.

Smith, J. W.: Manual of Medical Therapeutics. ed. 19. Boston, Little, Brown and Co., 1969.

14 IN-SERVICE EDUCATION

The accomplishment of intensive care for the patient who has suffered a myocardial infarction is dependent upon four interrelated factors:

1. A well-planned unit
2. Equipment
3. Personnel
4. A continuing educational program

The first two factors have been discussed in Chapters 4 and 5. We shall now consider the other two.

PERSONNEL

The coronary care unit is usually organized by the department of cardiology, which appoints a director to coordinate the program of care. His responsibilities include:

1. Establishing coronary care unit policies which have been developed by administration, the medical staff and nursing service
2. Developing an educational program for physicians and nurses
3. Setting and maintaining standards of care
4. Establishing techniques of care to treat the complications of myocardial infarction
5. Serving as liaison between the patient's physician and the coronary care unit personnel when problems arise

THE HOUSE STAFF

The medical resident assigned to the coronary care unit is likely to be the physician who will respond to any emergency calls concerning the patient's progress. In life-threatening situations he will direct the treatment and be responsible for its success or failure. Therefore, to insure the success of the unit, an educational program for physicians must be developed. This program should include:

1. An understanding of the intensive coronary care concept and the role of the nurse in this setting
2. Advanced study of the physiology of the circulatory system
3. A study of electrocardiography and recognition of arrhythmias
4. The pharmacology of drugs used in cardiac care
5. The recognition and treatment of the complications of myocardial infarction

EDUCATION OF THE PROFESSIONAL NURSE

The study program for the graduate nurse should be designed to give comprehensive training within a three- or four-week period. The course content should include lectures in:

1. Anatomy and physiology of the circulatory system
2. Diagnostic procedures
3. The development of coronary artery disease
4. Treatment of acute myocardial infarction
5. Philosophy of intensive coronary care
6. Psychological responses of the patient
7. Treatment of the complications of myocardial infarction
8. Treatment of the arrhythmias
9. Electrocardiography
10. Cardiac monitoring
11. Assisted respiration
12. Pharmacology of drugs used in cardiac care
13. Care of the patient with a pacemaker
14. Rehabilitation of the patient

The in-service instructor is responsible for implementing the intensive course. Participants should include:

1. A cardiologist
2. Medical resident
3. Anesthesiologist
4. Pharmacist
5. Nurse specialists

Class scheduling should be flexible in order to permit clinical observation of unusual events, such as cardiac arrest, insertion of a pacemaker catheter and so on.

The intensive course for the nurse is just the beginning of the educational process. To be considered fully prepared, a planned program of

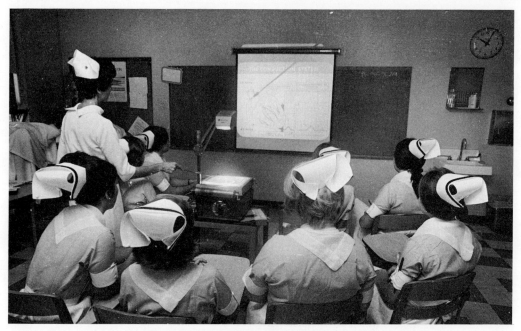

FIG. 14–1. Use of transparencies in teaching.

clinical experience must be set up in the coronary care unit which will permit the nurse to use all that she has learned. She should work a minimum of four months on days under close supervision of the head nurse.

In-service education should be continued on a weekly basis. Team conferences will augment the nurse's learning process. These conferences should be flexible in the utilization of various consulting personnel. The teaching personnel should fully understand the role of the nurse specialist.

A suggested pattern for a four-week intensive course in coronary care nursing could be as follows:

Pattern for a Four-Week Intensive Course

FIRST WEEK

Monday

8:00– 9:00	Philosophy and Concepts of Coronary Care
9:00–11:00	Anatomy and Physiology: Circulatory System
11:00–12:00	Diagnostic Procedures
1:00– 3:00	Basic Electrocardiography
3:00– 4:00	Atherosclerosis; Angina Pectoris

Tuesday

8:00–10:00	Anatomy and Physiology: Circulatory System
10:00–11:00	Diagnostic Procedures
11:00–12:00	Coronary Insufficiency; Coronary Occlusion
1:00– 3:00	Basic Electrocardiography
3:00– 4:00	Myocardial Infarction

Wednesday

8:00–10:00	Anatomy and Physiology: Circulatory System
10:00–12:00	Location of Infarctions
1:00– 3:00	Basic Electrocardiography
3:00– 4:00	Tour of the Coronary Care Unit

Thursday

8:00–10:00	Anatomy and Physiology: Respiratory System
10:00–12:00	Pharmacology: Cardiac Glycosides
1:00– 3:00	Basic Electrocardiography
3:00– 4:00	Admission of Patient to the Coronary Care Unit

Friday

8:00–10:00	Anatomy and Physiology: Respiratory System
10:00–12:00	Pharmacology: Diuretics
1:00– 3:00	Basic Electrocardiography
3:00– 4:00	Principles of Cardiac Monitoring

SECOND WEEK

Monday

8:00–10:00	Assisting With Care of a Patient and With Placement of Electrodes
10:00–12:00	Pharmacology: Vasoconstrictors
1:00– 2:00	Nurse–Patient Relationships
2:00– 3:00	Reaction to the Illness
3:00– 4:00	Reaction to the Environment

Tuesday

8:00–10:00	Assisting With Care of a Patient and ECG Lead Placement
10:00–12:00	Pharmacology: Vasoconstrictors
1:00– 2:00	Reaction to Discharge
2:00– 4:00	Left and Right Heart Failure

Wednesday

8:00–10:00	Assist With Care of a Patient; Run ECG Rhythm Strip
10:00–12:00	Pharmacology: Anticoagulants
1:00– 2:00	Rotating Tourniquets
2:00– 4:00	Cardiogenic Shock

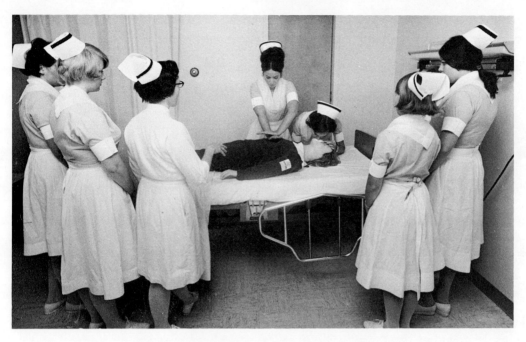

Fig. 14–2. Practicing cardiopulmonary resuscitation.

Thursday

8:00–10:00	Care of a Patient
10:00–11:00	Cardiac Arrhythmias
11:00–12:00	Premature Beats
1:00– 2:00	Sinus Arrhythmia
2:00– 3:00	Sinus Bradycardia
3:00– 4:00	Sinus Tachycardia

Friday

8:00–10:00	Care of a Patient
10:00–11:00	Atrial Tachycardia
11:00–12:00	Wandering Pacemaker
1:00– 2:00	Atrial Flutter
2:00– 3:00	Atrial Fibrillation
3:00– 4:00	Conference—Discussion of a Patient

THIRD WEEK

Monday

8:00–12:00	Care of a Patient
1:00– 3:00	Pharmacology: Antiarrhythmic Drugs
3:00– 4:00	Oxygen Therapy

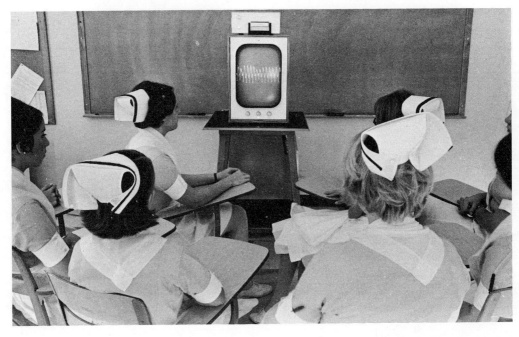

Fig. 14–3. Audiovisual training system for recognition of arrhythmias.

Tuesday

8:00–12:00	Care of a Patient
1:00– 2:00	Pulmonary Embolism
2:00– 4:00	Cardiac Arrest and Principles of Resuscitation

Wednesday

8:00–12:00	Care of a Patient
1:00– 4:00	Principles of Cardioversion; Demonstration and Use of the Defibrillator

Thursday

8:00–12:00	Care of a Patient
1:00– 2:00	Atrial Standstill
2:00– 4:00	Conference—Discussion of a Patient

Friday

8:00–12:00	Care of a Patient
1:00– 2:00	Ventricular Tachycardia
2:00– 4:00	Conference—Discussion of a Patient

FOURTH WEEK

Monday

8:00–12:00	Care of a Patient
1:00– 2:00	Ventricular Fibrillation
2:00– 4:00	Conference—Discussion of a Patient

Tuesday

8:00–12:00	Care of a Patient
1:00– 2:00	Ventricular Standstill
2:00– 3:00	Role of Electrolytes in ECG Changes
3:00– 4:00	Conference—Discussion of a Patient

Wednesday

8:00–12:00	Care of a Patient
1:00– 3:00	A-V Block; Left Bundle Branch Block; Right Bundle Branch Block
3:00– 4:00	Conference—Discussion of a Patient

Thursday

8:00–12:00	Care of a Patient
1:00– 2:00	Technique of External Pacing
2:00– 3:00	Temporary Pacing and Nursing Care
3:00– 4:00	Permanent Pacing and Nursing Care

Friday

8:00–12:00	Care of a Patient
1:00– 3:00	Rehabilitation
3:00– 4:00	Legal Aspects

TEACHING MATERIALS

1. Arrhythmia Resusci-Anne or Resusci-Anne
2. Audiovisual training system for recognition of cardiac arrhythmias
3. ECG rhythm strips (from unit file)
4. Emergency equipment
5. Monitoring equipment
6. Movie projector
7. Overhead projector
8. Transparency Series, "The Patient and Circulatory Disorders," Units I, II, III, Philadelphia, J. B. Lippincott Company, 1970

CORONARY CARE UNIT LIBRARY

Bernreiter, M.: Electrocardiography. ed. 2. Philadelphia, J. B. Lippincott, 1963.

Bordicks, K.: Patterns of Shock. New York, Macmillan, 1965.

Burch, G. E., and Winsor, T.: A Primer of Electrocardiography. ed. 5. Philadelphia, Lea & Febiger, 1966.

Corday, E., and Irving, D. W.: Disturbances of Heart Rate, Rhythm, and Conduction. ed. 2. Philadelphia, W. B. Saunders, 1962.

Goldman, M. J.: Principles of Clinical Electrocardiography. ed. 6. Los Altos, California, Lange Medical Publications, 1967.

Guyton, A. C.: Textbook of Medical Physiology. ed. 3. Philadelphia, W. B. Saunders, 1968.

Methany, N., and Snively, W. D.: Nurses' Handbook of Fluid Balance. Philadelphia, J. B. Lippincott, 1966.

Ritota, M.: Diagnostic Electrocardiography. Philadelphia, J. B. Lippincott, 1969.

Rodman, M. J., and Smith, D. W.: Pharmacology and Drug Therapy in Nursing. Philadelphia, J. B. Lippincott, 1968.

Shafer, K. N., Sawyer, J. R., McClusky, A. M., and Beck, E. C.: Medical-Surgical Nursing. ed. 4. St. Louis, C. V. Mosby, 1967.

Smith, D. W., and Gips, C. D.: Care of the Adult Patient. ed. 2. Philadelphia, J. B. Lippincott, 1966.

Wood, P.: Diseases of the Heart and Circulation. ed. 3. Philadelphia, J. B. Lippincott, 1968.

GLOSSARY

aberrant. Straying or wandering from the normal course.

acetylcholine. A choline ester which is important in the chemistry of the nerve impulse.

acidosis. A disturbance in the acid-base balance of the body due to an abnormal accumulation of acids or excessive loss of alkaline salts.

Adams-Stokes syndrome. A sudden attack of weakness and syncope due to cerebral ischemia. It occurs in complete heart block if the idioventricular pacemaker fails to control ventricular contraction.

adjustment. The process of coping with the internal and external environmental demands by means of some personal response.

aggression. A personal response that seeks the reduction of tension by means of behavior that is forceful, demanding or possessive.

alkalosis. An abnormal increase of alkaline substances in the body.

ampere. One ampere is produced by one volt acting through the resistance of one ohm, a unit of electrical current equivalent to one coulomb per second.

anastomosis. A union or communication between two normally separated vessels, fibers or parts of organs.

anger. A strong feeling of displeasure often involving a tendency to attack the object of displeasure.

angina pectoris. A clinical syndrome characterized by oppression and paroxysms of substernal pain. The pain may radiate to the neck and left arm.

anion. A negatively charged ion. The chief body anions are chloride, bicarbonate, phosphate.

anode. The positive electrode of an electric cell.

anoxemia. Diminution of oxygen supply in the blood.

anoxia. A deficient supply of oxygen to tissues.

anticoagulants. Drugs which decrease blood coagulation and which are used to prevent extension of clots and formation of emboli.

anxiety. Intense feelings of fearfulness and apprehension which stem from the anticipation of danger.

apathy. A marked absence of emotional sensitivity; emotional indifference in situations that normally move the emotions or interests.

arborization block. Delay or interruption of impulse transmission beyond the bundle branches in the Purkinje network.

arrhythmia. An irregular heart rhythm due to a disturbance in impulse formation, impulse conduction or both.

asynchronous. Lack of concurrence in time. Not occurring simultaneously.

asystole. Absence of heartbeat.

atherosclerosis. A disease of the arteries characterized by the development of fatty granulomatous lesions (atheromas) within or beneath the intimal surface of the vessel.

atrial fibrillation. A disturbance of impulse formation characterized by a rapid irregular rate ranging from 400–600 per minute.

atrial flutter. A disturbance in impulse formation characterized by a rapid atrial rhythm at the rate of 250–400 per minute.

atrial standstill. The absence of atrial activity for one or more beats, with the ventricles contracting in response to a secondary or tertiary pacemaker.

atrial tachycardia. A disturbance in impulse formation characterized by a rapid, regular rhythm with a heart rate above 140 beats per minute.

atrio-ventricular block. A delay or interruption of the electrical impulse through the A-V node.

first degree A-V block. A disturbance of impulse conduction in which the time of the impulse transmission to and through the A-V node is prolonged.

second degree A-V block. (See Wenckebach and Mobitz 2.)

third degree A-V block. A disturbance in impulse conduction in which the A-V node fails to conduct any impulses from the atria to the ventricles.

atrio-ventricular dissociation. A disturbance in impulse conduction in which the atria and ventricles are controlled by different pacemakers for one or more beats in the absence of antegrade block.

atrio-ventricular nodal rhythm. A disturbance of pacemaker function characterized by a slow pulse of 40–70 per minute. It is an escape rhythm in which a secondary pacemaker in the A-V node takes over by default of the S-A node.

automaticity. In heart cells, the property of regularly discharging an electrical impulse, and thus initiating contraction of the heart.

bigeminy. A pulse with a continuing rhythm characterized by two beats close together followed by a relatively long pause.

bradycardia. Abnormally slow heart rhythm of less than 60 beats per minute.

bundle branch block. A disturbance in impulse conduction in which the impulse from the S-A node is delayed or blocked through one of the bundle branches.

capture. To seize by force. In cardiology: to take control of the heartbeat by an ectopic pacemaker or electronic pacemaker.

cardiac arrest. Sudden cessation of the heartbeat, ventricular fibrillation in which the heartbeat is chaotic, or cardiovascular collapse in which the heartbeat is rhythmic, but ineffective. May manifest as ventricular asystole or total asystole.

cardiogenic shock. Shock caused by the inability of the heart to pump a sufficient amount of blood to all parts of the body. It is associated with a great decrease in cardiac output resulting from the impairment of myocardial contractility.

cardioversion. Use of the AC defibrillator to pass an electric current through the heart in order to stop an abnormal rhythm such as ventricular fibrillation.

cathode. The negative electrode of an electric cell.

cation. A positively charged ion. The chief body cations are sodium, potassium, calcium and magnesium.

collateral circulation. Small accessory blood vessels which anastomose when a main artery is occluded.

communication. The exchange of thoughts, ideas or messages by speech, gestures, expressions or writing.

compassion. To suffer with. Sharing the suffering of another by giving aid and support.

complex. Composed of two or more parts. In cardiology: the Q, R, S waves are called the QRS complex, which represents ventricular depolarization.

conduction block. Condition in which the propagation of the electrical impulse is delayed or stopped along its normal pathway.

conductivity. In heart cells, the property of transmitting electrical impulses, regardless of where the impulses originate.

coronary insufficiency. A clinical syndrome in which the cardiac pain is more prolonged than the pain of angina pectoris. An inadequate coronary blood flow for myocardial needs.

coronary occlusion. A blocking of a coronary artery which is caused by the formation of a blood clot in an atherosclerotic vessel.

coulomb. The quantity of electricity (equal to the charge in 6.25×10^{18} electrons) which is transferred in one second by one ampere.

denial. A defense mechanism used to relieve emotional conflict or anxiety, and characterized by a refusal to face or admit the reality of the disturbing factor or object.

depolarization. Loss of electrical charge.

diuretics. Agents which increase the flow of urine, and thus lead to the removal of the fluid of edema, and the excretion of sodium and other ions.

ectopic beat. Initiation of the cardiac cycle arising from a pacemaker other than the S-A node.

edema. The collection of excessive fluid in intercellular tissue spaces.

electrode. A conducting element in an electric cell or a semiconducting device.

electrolyte. A substance which, in solution, conducts electricity by means of ions.

electrophysiology. The study of the electromotive forces underlying various functions of the body. Electrocardiography (the recording of the moment-to-moment electrical energy or force generated by the heart during each cardiac cycle on a continuous time-voltage graph) is founded upon electrophysiological principles.

embolism. The obstruction of a blood vessel by a clot or other substance.

emotion. An affective response characterized by feeling, excitement and bodily change.

energy. The capacity or power to do work.

enzyme. Organic catalyst formed in living cells.

extrasystole. An interpolated premature heartbeat within a normal rhythm.

fusion beat. A joining together of two heartbeats due to a response of the atria or ventricles to two distinct impulses. Ventricular fusion beats are more common than atrial fusion beats.

galvanometer. An instrument which measures the direction and force of electrical current.

heart failure. A deficiency in cardiac output. In acute heart failure the deficiency in cardiac output occurs suddenly, intensely and rapidly. In chronic heart failure the deficiency in cardiac output is gradual and moderate in degree.

hemodynamics. Study of the principles and forces underlying the circulation of blood.

His, bundle of. The atrio-ventricular bundle, part of the conduction system in the heart.

hostility. An attitude or feeling involving aggressive behavior detrimental to individuals or groups against whom it is directed.

hypercalcemia. An excessive amount of calcium in the blood.

hyperkalemia. An excessive amount of potassium in the blood.

hypocalcemia. An abnormally low amount of calcium in the blood.

hypokalemia. An abnormally low amount of potassium in the blood.

hypoxemia. Lack of sufficient oxygen in the body cells.

idioventricular. Refers to the distinct function of the ventricle when dissociated from the atria.

idioventricular rhythm. A disturbance of pacemaker function characterized by a slow pulse of 30–35 per minute, which results from a slow ectopic impulse focused in the ventricles.

impulse. The product of a force or stimulus. In cardiology: refers to the electrical activity of the heart.

infarct. An area of tissue which undergoes necrosis due to deprivation of blood supply.

interference dissociation. A disturbance of impulse conduction occurring with A-V dissociation in which the ventricles beat faster than the atria. Occasionally, the atrial activation impulse discharges the A-V node prematurely and causes an interference beat. The slightly irregular rhythm which follows is called interference dissociation.

interpolated beat. An additional premature heartbeat inserted within a normal rhythm.

interval. A time lapse between two events. In electrocardiology: refers to the distance between recorded waves of the cardiac cycle.

intra-atrial block. A prolongation of the transmission time of the impulse conduction through atrial muscle.

inversion. An interchange of position of events occurring in a sequence. In electrocardiology: refers to the reversed positions of the P QRS T U waves.

ion. An electrically charged atom or group of atoms.

ischemia. Temporary lack of blood supply to tissue or an organ.

iso-electric. Having equal electrical potential. In electrocardiography it is recorded as a straight line.

lead. May refer to an electrocardiographic record or to one of the electrical attachments between the patient and the ECG machine.

magnetic field. A region or area in which a magnetic force can be detected.

milliequivalent. The chemical combining power of an ion equivalent to the chemical combining capacity of approximately one gram (atomic weight) of hydrogen.

Mobitz block, Type 2. Second degree heart block. A disturbance in impulse conduction in the A-V node in which there is a prolongation of the absolute refractory period.

monotopic. Refers to several premature beats arising from the same focus.

necrosis. Death of a specific area of tissue.

nodal tachycardia. A disturbance of impulse formation characterized by a regular, rapid pulse rate of 120–200 which occurs when the automaticity of the A-V node is enhanced above that of the S-A node, and the A-V node thus assumes the role of pacemaker.

occlusion. Obstruction or closing of a vessel.

ohm. In electricity a unit of resistance. A current of one ampere is prolonged when an electrical potential of one volt encounters a resistance of one ohm.

orthograde conduction. Propagation of the cardiac impulse in a proper, correct or standard direction.

oscilloscope. An electronic instrument that produces an instantaneous visual display of electric waves or motion on a screen of a cathode-ray tube.

osmosis. The passage of a solvent (usually water) from a region of a less concentrated solution, through a semipermeable membrane, to a region of a more concentrated solution, thereby tending to the equalization of the concentration of the two solutions.

pacemaker. Refers to the S-A node where the stimulus for the heartbeat normally originates.

palpitation. A rapid, forceful, throbbing pulsation of the heart.

paroxysmal. Sudden attack or recurrence of symptoms of a disease.

perfusion. Permeation, saturation or bathing of tissue with fluid, e.g., blood.

permeability. The capacity of a membrane or other tissue to allow the passing through of a fluid or substance in solution.

pH. A symbol used to designate the hydrogen ion concentration. Also used to express the degree of acidity or alkalinity of blood.

phlebothrombosis. Clotting in a vein.

polarized. Refers to the resting phase of the atria and ventricles.

polymorphic. Occurring in several forms or shapes.

polytopic. Refers to premature beats arising from more than one ectopic focus.

potassium. The dominant cation of the intracellular fluid; symbolized by K.

premature atrial beat. A disturbance in impulse formation, characterized by a beat which occurs earlier than expected in the basic rhythm due to an irritable focus in the atria.

premature nodal beat. A heartbeat which occurs early due to a disturbance of pacemaker function. It arises from an ectopic focus in the A-V node. Sometimes called premature junctional beats.

premature ventricular beat. A disturbance of impulse formation characterized by a ventricular beat which occurs early in relation to the basic rhythm.

Purkinje fibers. Specialized muscle fibers lying beneath the endocardium, which are part of the impulse-conduction system.

reciprocal beat. A beat which occurs in nodal rhythm when atrial activation is so delayed that the ventricle is no longer refractory and hence responds to the returning nodal impulse.

refractory period. A stage during which cardiac tissue is resistant to restimulation during the peak of fast action potential.

rehabilitation. A return to the activities of normal daily living through education and therapy.

repolarization. A rebuilding of an electrical gradient across a cell membrane.

resuscitation. Treatment directed toward returning a patient to a conscious state.

retrograde. Moving in a backward position.

salvo. A rapid discharge of heartbeats occurring in a regular sequence.

security. Protection from threat; implies some degree of control over one's environment.

sino-atrial block. A disturbance of conduction from the S-A node, in which one or more heartbeats are skipped.

sinus arrest. A disturbance of pacemaker function in which vagal suppression or disease of the S-A node results in failure of the node to initiate an electrical impulse.

sinus arrhythmia. A common variation of normal sinus rhythm in which the rate alternately increases and decreases due to alterations of vagal tone.

sodium. The dominant cation of the extracellular fluid; symbolized by Na.

ST segment. Represents the early phase of cardiac repolarization. No electrical forces are evident during this time, therefore no wave forms appear in the ECG.

supraventricular. Usually used to denote those areas above the bifurcation of the bundle of His (A-V bundle).

synchronize. To occur simultaneously; to operate in unison.

syncope. Loss of consciousness due to a temporary deficiency of cerebral blood supply.

tachycardia. An abnormally rapid heartbeat.

thrombus. A blood clot obstructing a vessel.

transaminase. An enzyme found in the heart, liver, muscle, kidneys and pancreas. Injury to one of these organs releases the transaminase from the damaged cell into the blood serum. Its presence, detected by laboratory analysis, is useful to confirm the diagnosis of myocardial infarction.

trigeminy. A pulse with a continuing rhythm characterized by three beats close together followed by a relatively long pause.

Valsalva maneuver. A test to determine early left ventricular failure by forced expiration against the closed glottis, which results in reduced venous pressure and a drop in arterial pressure.

vasopressor. A drug which constricts or narrows the blood vessels and thus raises the blood pressure.

vector. A force having magnitude and direction. Velocity is a vector embodying speed and direction of motion.

venous pressure. The pressure blood exerts within the veins. It indicates the heart's ability to handle the returning venous blood.

ventilate. The inspiration and expiration of air from the lungs.

ventricular fibrillation. A catastrophic arrhythmia characterized by rapid, ineffective, irregular and chaotic twitchings of the ventricles due to a rapid discharge of impulses focused in the ventricles. Circulation ceases because the ventricles do not contract.

ventricular standstill (ventricular asystole). Absence of ventricular contraction.

ventricular tachycardia. A disturbance of impulse formation characterized by a rapid, almost regular ventricular rate of 150–200 beats per minute due to a ventricular ectopic focus.

volt. The unit of electromotive force required to produce one ampere of current through a resistance of one ohm.

voltage. Electromotive force or potential expressed in volts.

wandering pacemaker. A disturbance of pacemaker functions in which the pacemaker wanders back and forth from the S-A node to the A-V node, and which is characterized by slight variations in cardiac rhythm.

Wenckebach block. A type of second degree heart block in which the P-R interval increases progressively until a QRS complex is omitted after which the P-R interval becomes smaller. The event recurs in a series of successive cycles.

INDEX